D1881398

SPORTS MEDICINE AND EXERCISE SCIENCE

SPORTS MEDICINE AND EXERCISE SCIENCE

Editor
G.C. Satpathy

ISHA BOOKS
DELHI-110 033

Sports Medicine and Exercise Science

Rs. 890

ISBN: 81-8205-148-7

© G.C. Satpathy

All rights reserved. No part of this book may be reproduced in any manner without written permission.

Published in 2005 in India by
Isha Books, D-43, Prithviraj Road,
Adarsh Nagar, Delhi-110 033

Laser Typesetting at : Shree Vaishnavi Creations, Delhi
Printed at : Chawla Offset Press, Delhi

Contents

Preface

Sports medicine is a new and exciting medical discipline charged with the care of the injured and sick athletes. It is a multidisciplinary field involving many facets of the health care community. In many countries it has become an independent speciality with its own colleges and associations; nevertheless its charge crosses the disciplines of orthopaedics, rehabilitation medicine, nutrition, psychiatry, emergency medicine, paediatrics, geriatrics, gynaecology, dermatology and primary care.

Exercise is one of the major component of sports medicine. The purpose of exercise is to stress systematically the body so it improves its capacity to exercise. The benefits of regular exercise are now well established for all groups in the community including the young, old, disabled and the unwell. There are countless exercise devices and training programs available that are hailed as the best way to gain strength. For most sports, training probably has a greater effect on performance than nutrition, equipment, psychological state, or any other modifiable factor. Training can also cause injuries, and over-training can lead to illness. The quantification or measurement of training is therefore an important issue for athletes, coaches, and sport scientists.

The present volume provides authentic information of sports medicine and exercise practices which each sportsperson should be aware of. It gives essential guidelines for physicians and trainers of sportperson to provide appropriate care and treatment. Sports personalities, sports medicine specialists, team physicians, coaches, trainers and budding student-athletes will find this work highly informative and useful. It will equip the reader with a state of the art knowledge of sports medicine and exercise science.

Editor

1

Competitive Sports Training

For most sports, training probably has a greater effect on performance than nutrition, equipment, psychological state, or any other modifiable factor. Training can also cause injuries, and overtraining can lead to illness. The quantification or measurement of training is therefore an important issue for athletes, coaches, and sport scientists.

Characteristics of Training

Training is a complex behavior, mainly because it is performed in a time frame that ranges from seconds to years. Sportspeople use numerous terms to describe the characteristics of this temporal dimension of training. Single human movements, which occur in a second or two, are combined and repeated to make a training bout or workout, a period of more-or-less uninterrupted physical activity. Workouts may occupy a few minutes or hours, and may be continuous exercise, a set of reps or repeated movements, or a set of sets. A complete training session usually lasts an hour or two and consists of one or more workouts. The nature of each session may vary, but after a week or so a repeated pattern of sessions known as a microcycle usually emerges. A series of microcycles may constitute a phase of training, for example a build-up or speciality phase. A repeated pattern of phases or microcycles makes up a mesocycle, and a season or macrocycle of training may consist of a repeated set of mesocycles. Finally, over a period of years a training history develops. Studies involving quantification of training focus invariably on only a small part of the training time frame.

In some biomechanical applications, the focus of interest is a single movement or limited set of movements, such as a high jump or a javelin throw. In most other applications, particularly those involving investigation of the physiological effects of training, the fundamental unit of training is the workout. Even in studies of injury and illness that focus on a season or history of training, data on typical workouts during one or more phases of training usually provide the key training variables. Workouts vary between sports, but most can be classified as either endurance, interval, strength or skill. For example, in competitive track running a workout of continuous running is classified as endurance; repetition running (short periods of high-speed running separated by rests or slow-speed running) is an example of an interval workout; short sprints with a weight in tow qualifies as a strength workout; and practicing of starts is a skill workout.

This classification reflects common usage by sportspeople, but it also has an underlying theoretical basis: in general, endurance workouts train the aerobic power system, interval workouts train the anaerobic glycolytic system, strength workouts train the phosphagen system, and skill workouts train the central nervous system.

Duration and intensity are important characteristics of a training workout, because they contribute to the short- and long-term effects of the workout on the health and fitness of the athlete. In the case of an endurance workout performed at a reasonably steady pace, only one estimate of duration and intensity may be required. Interval and strength workouts involve multiple periods of work and rest, each of which may need an estimate of intensity and duration. The intensity and duration of skill workouts also need to be characterized, especially if the movements are practiced at sufficiently high intensity and for a sufficient duration to produce a training effect on the body's power systems. The aims of a study will dictate whether other aspects of training workouts need to be assayed. For example, it may be important to determine details of clothing, equipment, training surface or medium, venue, time of day, weather, consumption of food or drink, psychological state, supervision, or perhaps even the number and caliber of training companions.

Methods of Quantification

There are three groups of methods:

i) observational (taking measurements in real time or from video recordings),

ii) physiological (monitoring heart rate, blood lactate concentration or oxygen consumption), and

ii) subjective (use of questionnaires or diaries).

The methods in each group are similar in their suitability for assaying training, but there are substantial differences between groups.

Observational methods

Quantification of periods of training from a few seconds to a few weeks can be achieved simply by observing the training either in real time or on video. Practical considerations set the upper limit of the time frame: it is time-consuming for the coach or scientist to be present at every training session, and expensive if observers or video operators are employed. Observation may also cause the athletes to train more intensely or closer to their prescription than they would otherwise do, but in general the measures obtained by observation are probably more valid than those obtained by physiological or subjective means.

Real-time observation

The measures usually recorded in real time are the type and duration of the workout, along with relevant split times, distances, weights or workloads that produce measures of intensity. Special stopwatches facilitate recording of multiple times if the workout is a set of intervals. Information on other dimensions such as weather and equipment is also recorded if relevant. It is worth making a recording form with coded columns for all the necessary data. Such forms reduce the rates of error and loss of data and can be sent directly to a data-capture service.

Measures of intensity derived from observation can be expressed either in absolute terms (e.g., pace in minutes per mile) or in relative terms (e.g., pace as a percent of the athlete's personal best pace for the distance). For athletes doing resistance training with weights, an important measure of relative intensity is the repetitions maximum (RM); for example, 80% of 1 RM is 80% of the weight that an athlete can only just lift once. The use of relative intensity simplifies description or prescription of intensity for athletes who differ in ability.

Video

Video is a tool primarily for the coach or biomechanist interested in improving the athlete's skill. It is ideal for the analysis of single movements or intervals of exercise lasting up to a minute or two. The most cost-effective method is qualitative analysis, in which the athlete, coach or sport scientist simply view the video together and decide immediately how technique could be improved. The athlete can then attempt any recommended changes and be filmed for a further round of analysis.

Quantitative analysis involves digitization of the video images to permit calculation of spatial and temporal relationships in the movement. Several proprietary hardware-software packages are available for the purpose. Simple but effective digitizing is also possible with minimal extra hardware and software. The procedure is time-consuming and loses the benefit of immediate feedback to the athlete, but it allows detailed comparisons of one athlete with another or of one athlete before and after an intervention. Video has also been used for time-motion or notational analysis, in which the times spent in various modes of activity or in moving at various speeds are estimated from time and distance measurements taken from the video. As yet the method has been employed only for quantification of the energy demands of competition rather than of training.

Physiological methods

Training produces many effects on the body, ranging from acute responses (e.g., increase in breathing frequency during exercise) to chronic adaptations (e.g., increase in blood volume and maximum oxygen consumption after a few weeks of endurance training). Some chronic adaptations find application in studies of the training of non-athletes, where they can provide objective evidence of an increase in physical activity. With athletes, only the acute responses are used to quantify training, and of these responses only three have any practical significance: oxygen consumption, heart rate, and blood lactate concentration. All three provide information only on the intensity of steady-state exercise.

The need for special apparatus to monitor physiological responses sets the upper limits on the useful time frame for these methods. Devices are now available that will allow athletes to monitor their own heart rates indefinitely, but if the data are to be collected by a researcher, several months of monitoring is difficult to achieve. Measurement of lactate concentration is also difficult to sustain for more than a few months, while oxygen consumption requires equipment that can be used realistically only for a few training sessions. The shortest duration of training that can be monitored is set by the response time of the physiological variables to changes in exercise intensity. Oxygen consumption and heart rate take 3-4 min to reach a steady state, and blood lactate concentration takes even longer, so these variables are unable to provide readily interpretable information on the intensity of reps/intervals.

Oxygen consumption

In theory this is a good measure of the intensity of steady-state exercise, for a number of reasons.

— Training that can be sustained at a constant pace for more than a few minutes is performed with energy supplied almost entirely from consumption of oxygen.

— The relationship between steady-state oxygen consumption and power output or speed is linear over the range of intensity from rest to maximum steady state.

— Oxygen consumption drifts upwards by only a few percent in prolonged exercise performed at a constant high workload.

— Oxygen consumption at a given workload is stable over a period of months of training, in part because exercise efficiency changes little in trained athletes.

In practice, measurement of oxygen consumption requires athletes to breathe into special apparatus to allow expired gas to be collected or analyzed. This requirement limits the monitoring of training activities in the field, although several portable devices weighing only a few kilograms are now available. It is more convenient (but less representative of real training) if the activity can be performed in a laboratory on a sport-specific ergometer. Analysis of oxygen consumption is possible in real time with one of a range of available metabolic carts or with a similar computerized system of analyzers of gas volume and composition; alternatively, Douglas bags can be used to store the gas for later analysis. If analyzing or collecting gas is too difficult during the training activity, it is possible to analyze or collect gas for several minutes immediately after the activity, then to calculate the oxygen consumption that occurred during the activity by back-extrapolation.

Several measures of intensity can be derived from oxygen consumption. Of the absolute measures, milliliters of oxygen per minute per kilogram of body mass ($ml.min^{-1}.kg^{-1}$) is appropriate for comparing training that involves continual changes in direction or speed, or continuous work against gravity (examples: running, off-road cycling, most team sports). Liters of oxygen per minute ($L.min^{-1}$) is better for sports like road cycling and swimming. A relative measure that is rarely, if ever, used with athletes is the met (multiple of the resting metabolic rate). The most common relative measure is oxygen consumption expressed as a percent of maximum oxygen consumption, which is usually determined in an incremental test to maximum effort with the same mode of exercise as the training activity. The relative oxygen consumption allows more meaningful comparison of the training intensities of athletes who differ in body mass, performing ability, and exercise efficiency. For reasons already stated, it is not possible to measure the intensity of short intervals of high-intensity training directly as an oxygen consumption. It is nevertheless possible to exploit the linear relationship between workload (or pace) and oxygen consumption to express the intensity of such workouts as a percent of maximum oxygen consumption. For this purpose the oxygen consumption of several steady-state workouts is determined and plotted against workload, the line through the points is extrapolated to the higher workloads of the interval training, and the "corresponding" oxygen consumption is read off the graph.

Heart rate

This variable shows a response to exercise similar to that of oxygen consumption, so it can be used in a similar fashion to measure intensity when work load is maintained reasonably constant for more than a few minutes. Heart rate is higher if the same exercise is performed in a hotter environment. It also drifts upward more than oxygen consumption as the athlete heats up in prolonged exercise. It has the advantage over oxygen consumption of being far easier to assay.

In the laboratory heart rates are usually measured with an electrocardiograph, but for field work a range of miniaturized cardiotachometers is available. The most reliable of these detect the electrical activity of the heart and use it to calculate heart rate. Models that store the heart rate allow the coach and sport scientist to make use of the data, which are either replayed on the watch or downloaded into a computer or special portable analyzing unit. Waterproof versions can be used to monitor steady-state aquatic training. The athlete can also measure heart rate directly by palpation of an artery in the wrist or neck, but exercise has to be stopped briefly to perform the measurement and the resulting estimate is not accurate.

Heart rate can be used to express intensity in several ways. The absolute heart rate is useful for the individual athlete monitoring intensity on a day-to-day basis. Heart rate expressed as a percent of maximum controls for differences in the maximum heart rate between athletes.

Differences in the resting heart rate can be taken into account if intensity is expressed as a percent of heart-rate reserve: 100(training heart rate - resting heart rate)/(maximum heart rate - resting heart rate). A practical method of specifying intensity is to express training heart rates as a percent of race-pace heart rate. Heart rate recorded in the field can also be converted to oxygen consumption or other measure of training pace or power using relationships between heart rate and pace derived for each athlete from a series of steady-state exercise tests.

Lactate concentration

During intense exercise lactate produced in muscle by the anaerobic glycolytic pathway diffuses into the blood and causes the blood lactate concentration to rise above the resting value 1-2 mmol.L^{-1}. If the intensity is not too high, blood lactate reaches a steady level after 10-20 min of steady exercise. The relationship between the steady level of lactate and workload is curvilinear but reproducible, which means that lactate can be used to define training intensity. The range of intensities over which this method works is narrow: moderate intensities do not evoke increases in blood lactate, and at high intensities lactate does not reach a steady value before the athlete fatigues.

The highest intensity at which lactate stabilizes is one definition of the anaerobic threshold, and it corresponds to a blood lactate concentration of about 4 mmol.L^{-1}.

Exercise at this intensity can be sustained for 30-60 min before fatigue occurs. Blood lactates are measured during training mostly for determination of the anaerobic threshold, then for prescription of intensity of training relative to the threshold. The peak value of lactate concentration reached during or following short high-intensity workouts is sometimes measured by enthusiastic sportspeople, but this practice is not useful. Compact lactate analyzers are available for determination of blood lactate concentration in a droplet of blood taken from a finger or earlobe. A portable instrument, suitable for use in the field, is also available.

The analysis is rapid (1-2 min) and reliable, although technically demanding for the non-scientist. Problems with the technique arise not from the lactate analysis itself but from variability between athletes: the intensity corresponding to a blood lactate concentration of 4 $mmol.L^{-1}$ is perceived as moderate by some athletes and too hard to sustain by others. Even within the same athlete, variations in muscle glycogen content caused by recent training or diet can alter the lactate concentration corresponding to the anaerobic threshold. Care should therefore be taken to standardize training and diet for the few days before blood lactate is monitored.

Subjective methods

Questionnaires and diaries are closely related instruments: a diary is effectively a series of self-administered questionnaires. Both instruments obtain data recalled from memory, and both can be used to assay training over all but the shortest time frames.

Quantification of a behavior as complex as training is an exercise in simplification, which occurs at several stages. The most crucial simplification occurs when data are first recorded: if too much detail is sought, the athletes or the researcher will be overwhelmed; on the other hand, details lost at this stage may be important determinants of performance or health. Further simplification occurs at the stage of data analysis, when variables representing the raw training data are combined into one or more global measures of training to permit modeling of relationships between training and performance or health. Statistics should also be simplified and presented with as little jargon as possible, especially if the audience is athletes, coaches, or other lay people.

Statistical analysis of training data poses several challenges. Variables representing training duration or volume are usually not normally distributed, so they need to be transformed if they are the outcome variables in an analysis. Log transformation usually works well and has the bonus that outcomes can be represented as percent changes or percent differences in training. Rank transformation (resulting in non-parametric analysis) is a second-best choice.

Training affects the health and fitness of the athlete through duration and intensity, but combining these two variables into a single global measure of training is fraught with difficulty. The simplest and probably best approach is to multiply them together and add them up over all intensities. The resulting variable has the dimensions of work done or energy consumed in performing the exercise. It is sometimes known as a TRIMP (TRaining IMPulse). A problem with this variable is that training performed at a particular intensity for a particular duration produces the same TRIMP as training performed at twice the intensity for half the duration, yet training at the higher intensity usually has disproportionately greater effects on the body. Attempts to introduce a non-linear factor to make higher intensity training contribute more to the total TRIMP score should be avoided, because the value of the factor is arbitrary.

Measurement of training

The two groups of sports professionals who make use of methods to quantify training are practitioners (athletes and coaches) and scientists. For practitioners, the main applications are to motivate the athlete, make training systematic, and prescribe training. Sport scientists are interested in the relationships between training and performance, or between training and various aspects of the health of the athlete.

Use by sports practitioners

Motivation to adhere to training regimes is likely to be enhanced by any interest shown in the athlete's training, but the high-tech appeal of physiological monitoring and video recording probably succeeds more in this respect than other methods. Diaries appear to be the best way to promote systemization of training behavior, through their ability to produce a continuous record of training; the process of reviewing the training data in a diary should also stimulate a critical approach to the purpose of duration, intensity and skill components of specific workouts and to the purpose of the periodized structure in the training program.

Diaries are the most effective method for checking whether most aspects of a training prescription are being followed, provided the coach can be confident about the athlete's honesty or accuracy. Prescribed targets of training intensity for steady-state exercise can be set and checked with heart rate monitoring; lactate monitoring has also been promoted for this purpose, but it is probably not reliable or practical enough for the coach or athlete.

Use by sport scientists

The research interests of sport scientists fall into two groups: performance and health. The majority of researchers in both groups have used questionnaires as the main method of quantifying training, especially for descriptive studies. Experimental studies, in which the effects of an imposed change in training have been investigated, have been conducted mainly over short periods of time and have used mainly real-time observation to verify compliance with the training program. Past and present topics of interest in studies of training and performance have included the training behaviors of better performers, the effect of increasing the intensity of training, the effect of training or living at altitude on sea-level performance, and effect of a taper phase of training before a competition. Studies of the relationship between training and health of athletes have dealt with aspects of overtraining, injury, illness, wellness, immune function, psychological state, reproductive function and nutrition.

Sports medicine is concerned with the care and the potential performance of the athlete. It requires a comprehensive approach; unlike the fragmentation seen in technological medicine this century. These principles of care were established by Herodicus of Selymbria and Claudius Galen They emphasized training, diet, massage and a medical approach to athletics. Galen's contribution to scientific medicine was monumental. He placed the clinical instructions of Hippocrates on a sound experimental basis; for 1500 years his works dominated medical knowledge. He was a true sports medicine practitioner (the father of sports medicine). Pontifex Maximus made him physician to the gladiators in the

Pergamon arena in Asia Minor and he published his methods of treatment. It is well to set Galen's contribution among others.

Epidemiology is the medical discipline which deals with the occurrence, causes and prevention of disease. Its methodology, used in public health to study outbreaks of disease and to design preventive measures, is widely applied in sports medicine to injury rather than illness or disease. The epidemiological approach contributes much to better understanding of the incidence and causes of injuries and allows planning of prevention programs and the proper allocation of medical resources. An understanding of the implications of assumptions inherent in the statistical methods underlying epidemiological methods is necessary if some common pitfalls are to be avoided (e.g. no clear hypothesis under test, poor definition of injury type, inappropriate controls, population under study not defined, over-generalization of results). Snow skiing injuries have been extensively studied as has American football (because of the high incidence of head and spinal injuries). Interventional studies now being published examine the role of knee and ankle braces in injury prevention. With time more multi-centre studies will be planned to gather data on the effects of interventional measures.

Investigating sports injuries

Epidemiological approaches to sports injuries may be descriptive or analytical. Descriptive studies define the problem in terms of incidence and prevalence. Analytical studies seek to identify risk factors with the goal of doing something about the injury rate, or to evaluate the effectiveness of treatment regimes.

Incidence (rate) of injury is the number of cases per unit time. The rate of injury is measured as the number of injuries or injured athletes (note the significance of the distinction in relation to multiple injuries which may be of different type) over a specified period, and may be expressed in absolute or relative terms (e.g. 3.0 skiing injuries per 1000 skier days). The risk of injury (the probability that an individual will be injured) is measured in the exposed population as a cumulative incidence giving the proportion injured, by actuarial methods (difficult) or from incidence densities. These two parameters provide the basis for most studies of sports injuries.

Risk factors

Identification of risk factors provides a means for doing something about the sports injury problem. Both the observational and experimental approaches of analytical epidemiology are used. Observational study designs are of three main types are given:

1. *Case-control*—the injured group is compared with a non-injured group in relation to a potential risk factor. Such studies are retrospective, easy to conduct and commonly used, but careful matching of controls is important. The possible sources of bias, role of sampling vagaries and confounding variables must be carefully assessed.

2. *Cohort* —similar design, but prospective in that groups exposed or not exposed to a potential risk factor are recognized before injury and then followed through time. This approach is less susceptible to information bias. data collection takes longer and the method is more expensive to implement . Variations

include surveillance designs (continuous monitoring of a group of athletes as under the National Athlete Injury/Illness Reporting System in the USA or NEISS). In survival designs, survival curve analysis is used to follow the reduction in proportion of uninjured/injured over the study period (as in follow-up of orthopaedic joint replacement).

3. *Cross-sectional*—documents injuries and risk factors at one point in time, describing prevalence and injury patterns. This approach is of limited value where rehabilitation times after injury are long.

Experimental study designs are interventional. Subjects are assigned randomly to treatment or control groups (e.g. prophylactic wearing of ankle splints in basketball). Ethical problems may arise in relation to allocation/withholding of potentially useful treatment.

The effectiveness of treatment is best studied in randomized clinical trials which should be double blinded as compliance with protocol is otherwise difficult to achieve. The study plan covers selection of patients (inclusion and exclusion criteria must be clearly defined), random allocation of treatments, treatment and analysis.

Exercise and Metabolism

Knowledge of the biochemistry and physiology of exercise is essential for interpreting the complex reactions involved in physical exertion. This knowledge can be applied to improve not only the performance of athletes, but also to monitor the health of the exercising public and to improve some medical conditions. Exercise has beneficial metabolic effects relevant to many areas of medicine, such as in diabetes, in the prevention of atherosclerosis and obesity, and in the management of stress. Regular exercise lowers: the resting heart rate, blood pressure, diabetic insulin requirements, LDL (low density lipoprotein) and triglycerides, while it increases: HDL (high density lipoprotein) and lean body mass. With appropriate exercise, the cardiovascular capacity overall improves and the cardiovascular risk is lowered. In some medical conditions fatigue occurs after mild exertion e.g. peripheral vascular disease. From information based on the metabolism of exercise and the ensuring fatigue, assessment and treatment can be implemented through strategies such as suitable nutrition and training programs. In general genetic reproduction, adaptive capability, and metabolism maintain the human condition.

Cardiovascular response to exercise

During exercise, the cardiac output increases, enabling the cardiovascular system to increase the transport of oxygen to the working muscles and to remove the metabolic heat produced by transferring it to the skin surface for evaporation, while still maintaining the blood pressure to supply blood to the brain. Maximum exercise capacity is determined by increased O_2 delivery from increased cardiac stroke volume and so cardiac output (CO = SV x HR), vasodilatation and to a much lesser extent increased mitochondrial volume. Such capacity decreased with age from reduced max HR and reduced SV, although exercise may maintain it.

Pulmonary response to exercise

During exercise, the pulmonary ventilation also increases

in order to augment oxygen supplies to the exercising muscles and remove waste carbon dioxide from the increased oxidative metabolism. Exercise improves the efficiency of the respiratory muscles and increases the total lung capacity by reducing the residual volume. The vital capacity is increased and elite athletes have very large vital capacity. The maximum minute volume is also increased by athletic training and endurance athletes are able to process large volumes of air during competition.

2

Overhead Throwing Athlete

The repetitive microtraumatic stresses placed on the athlete's shoulder joint complex during the throwing motion challenge the physiologic limits of the surrounding tissues. Frequently, alterations in throwing mechanics, muscle fatigue, muscle weakness or imbalance, and excessive capsular laxity may lead to tissue breakdown and injury. These injuries frequently involve the glenohumeral capsule, glenoid labrum, and the rotator cuff musculature. It has been our experience that most injuries to the thrower's shoulder can be effectively treated with a proper nonoperative rehabilitation program.

Generally, the rehabilitation program consists of activity modification, flexibility exercises, strengthening exercises, and a gradual return to throwing activities. The rehabilitation program for each of the classifications. A classification system for injuries to the thrower's shoulder. Each of these abnormalities develops because of unique etiologic factors. On the basis of these etiologic factors and the clinical examination, a proper rehabilitation program can be developed for each category. The key to effective treatment is a thorough clinical examination and appropriate differential diagnosis.

Before the specifics of the rehabilitation program can be discussed, a thorough understanding of the clinical examination of the shoulder joint complex must be established. The evaluation of the thrower's shoulder has been discussed in part two of the series. The physician must evaluate the thrower to establish a differential diagnosis, then the physical therapist or athlete trainer must evaluate the thrower to establish a list of physical limitations or problems that may be contributing to or resulting from the disorder.

The rehabilitation specialist must evaluate range of motion, muscle strength, laxity, and proprioception. In addition, the rehabilitation specialist should address the athlete's throwing program, exercise schedule, and throwing mechanics. Once these areas have been assessed, a comprehensive rehabilitation program can be established. Furthermore, during the evaluation process, the clinician must have an understanding of what is considered to be the "normal" or acceptable physiologic characteristics for the overhead throwing population. The purpose of the following sections is to convey to the reader the typical physical characteristics of the overhead throwing athlete. Specific range of motion, strength, laxity, and proprioceptive characteristics exhibited in throwing athletes will be discussed. The clinician must possess a complete understanding of what is typical for this unique athletic population so that abnormalities or differences can be appropriately identified and addressed.

Range of motion

Most throwers exhibit an obvious motion disparity

whereby external rotation is excessive and internal rotation is limited at 90° of abduction. Several investigators have documented that pitchers exhibit greater external rotation of the shoulder than do position players. Some reported that professional pitchers exhibited 141° ± 15° of shoulder external rotation measured at 90° of abduction. This was approximately 9° more than the nonthrowing shoulder, and approximately 9° more than the throwing shoulder of position players measured in 90° of abduction.

The investigators reported that the pitchers' external rotation at 90° of abduction averaged 118° (range, 95° to 145°) in the dominant shoulder, whereas the position players' dominant shoulder averaged 108° (range, 80° to 105°). In an ongoing study of professional baseball players, assessed the range of shoulder motion of 372 professional baseball players. The pitchers exhibit an average of 129.9° ± 10° of external rotation and 62.6°±9° of internal rotation when passively assessed at 90° of abduction.

In pitchers, the external rotation is approximately 7° greater in the throwing shoulder when compared with the nonthrowing shoulder, while internal rotation is 7° greater in the nonthrowing shoulder. In addition, the total motion (external rotation and internal rotation added together) in the throwing shoulder is equal (within 5°) when compared with the nonthrowing shoulder. This was consistent in all 372 baseball players. The "total motion concept". The pitchers exhibit the greatest total arc of motion; that is, external and internal rotation at 90° of abduction, followed closely by catchers, then outfielders, and finally infielders. Furthermore, when comparing left-handed with right-handed pitchers, the left-handed throwers exhibit approximately 7° more external rotation and 12° more total motion when compared with right-handed throwers. These findings were statistically significant.

Laxity

Most throwers exhibit significant laxity of the glenohumeral joint, which permits excessive range of motion. The hypermobility of the thrower's shoulder has been referred to as "thrower's laxity." The laxity of the anterior and inferior glenohumeral joint capsule may be appreciated by the clinician during the stability assessment of the overhead thrower's shoulder joint. Some clinicians have reported that the excessive laxity exhibited by the thrower is the result of repetitive throwing and they have referred to this as "acquired laxity", while others have documented that the overhead thrower exhibits congenital laxity.

The investigators noted a high degree of inferior glenohumeral joint laxity, with 61% of pitchers and 47% of position players exhibiting a positive sulcus sign in the throwing shoulder. Additionally, in the players who also exhibited a positive sulcus sign in the dominant shoulder, 89% of the pitchers and 100% of the position players exhibited a positive sulcus sign in the nondominant shoulder. Thus, it would appear that some baseball players exhibit inherent or congenital laxity, with superimposed acquired laxity, as a result of adaptive changes from throwing.

Muscle strength

Several investigators have examined muscle strength parametersin the overhead throwing athlete with varying results and conclusions. The investigators demonstrated that the external rotation strength of the pitcher's throwing shoulder is significantly weaker than the nonthrowing shoulder, by 6%. Conversely, internal rotation strength of the throwing shoulder was significantly stronger, by 3%, compared with the nonthrowing shoulder. In addition, adduction strength of the throwing shoulder is also significantly stronger than in the nonthrowing shoulder, by approximately 9% to 10%. The important isokinetic value is the unilateral muscle ratio, which describes the antagonist/agonist muscle strength ratio.

A proper balance between agonist and antagonist muscle groups is thought to provide dynamic stabilization to the shoulder joint. To provide proper muscle balance, a Data condensed from Wilk et al. the external rotator muscles should be at least 65% the strength of the internal rotator muscles. Optimally, the external-to-internal rotator muscles strength ratio should be 66% to 75%. This provides proper muscle balance.

Table 1 illustrates the expected muscle strength values of professional baseball players. In pitchers, the supraspinatus muscle was significantly weaker on the throwing side compared with the nonthrowing side; this was tested by performing an isometric manual muscle test of the empty can maneuver. Additionally, pitchers were weaker than the control group of nonbaseball players for shoulder abduction, external rotation, internal rotation, and muscle strength of the supraspinatus muscle. The scapular muscles play a vital role during the overhead throwing motion. Proper scapular movement and stability are imperative for asymptomatic shoulder function. These muscles work in a synchronized fashion and act as force couples about the scapula, providing both movement and stabilization. Wilk et al. documented the isometric scapular muscle strength values of professional baseball players.

The results indicated that pitchers and catchers exhibited a significantly different strength increase of the protractor and elevator muscles of the scapula when compared with position players.

All players (except infielders) exhibited significantly stronger depressor muscles of the scapula on the throwing side compared with the nonthrowing side. In addition, the agonist/antagonist muscle ratios are important values when considering how the scapula provides stability, mobility, and symptom-free function. Table 2 illustrates the scapular muscle strength values in the overhead throwing athlete.

Table 1

Glenohumeral Muscular Strength Values (in percent) in Professional Baseball Playersa

	180 deg/s	*300 deg/s*	*450 deg/s*
Bilateral comparisons			
External rotation	95-109	85-95	80-80
Internal rotation	105-120	100-115	100-110
Abduction	100-110	100-110	
Adduction	120-135	115-130	
Unilateral muscle ratios			
External/internal rotation	63-70	65-72	62-70
Abduction/adduction	82-87	92-97	
External rotation/abduction	64-69	66-71	
Isokinetic torque/body weight ratios			
External rotation	18-23	15-20	
Internal rotation	27-33	25-30	
Abduction	26-32	20-26	
Adduction	32-36	28-33	

Proprioception

Proprioception is defined as the conscious or unconscious awareness of joint position, whereas neuromuscular control is the efferent motor response to afferent (sensory) information. The thrower relies on enhanced proprioception to influence the neuromuscular system to dynamically stabilize the glenohumeral joint in the presence of significant capsular laxity and excessive range of motion. Allegrucci et al. tested the shoulder proprioception in 20 healthy overhead throwing athletes participating in various sports. Testing of joint proprioception was performed on a motorized system with the subject attempting to reproduce a specific joint angle.

The investigators noted that the dominant shoulder exhibited diminished proprioception compared with the nondominant shoulder. The investigators also noted improved proprioception near the end range of motion when compared with the starting point. Some reported that, in persons with clinically determined generalized joint laxity, the laxity is significantly less sensitive during proprioceptive testing. The proprioceptive capability of 120 professional baseball players. The investigators passively positioned the player's arm at a documented point within the player's external rotation range of motion.

The athlete was then instructed to actively reposition the shoulder in the same position. The researchers noted no significant difference between the throwing shoulder and nonthrowing shoulder. In addition, Wilk et al. compared the proprioceptive ability of 60 professional baseball players with that of 60 nonoverhead throwing athletes. The investigators noted no significant differences between baseball players and the others. However, baseball players exhibited slightly improved proprioceptive abilities at external rotation end range of motion compared with nonoverhead athletes, but these results were not significantly different.

Rehabilitation Programme for the Overhead Thrower

The nonoperative rehabilitation program used for treatment of shoulder injuries to the overhead thrower involves a multiphased approach that is progressive and sequential. The specific goals of each of the four phases of the program are outlined in Table 2. Each phase represents a progression from the prior phase: the exercises become more aggressive and demanding, and the stresses applied to the shoulder joint gradually increase. The the specific rehabilitation exercises and drills that use to treat the overhead throwing athlete. There are 10 rehabilitation principles that follow when treating a throwing athlete. These principles are shown in Table 3.

Table 2

Rehabilitation of the Overhead Thrower—Phases and Goals

Phase one—acute phase
Goals
- Diminish pain and inflammation
- Normalize motion
- Retard muscular atrophy
- Reestablish dynamic stability (muscular balance)
- Control functional stress/strain

Exercises and modalities:
- Cryotherapy, ultrasound, electrical stimulation
- Flexibility and stretching for posterior shoulder muscles (improve internal rotation and horizontal adduction)

(Contd...)

(Contd...)

Rotator cuff strengthening (especially external rotator muscles)
Scapular muscles strengthening (especially retractor, protractor, depressor muscles)
Dynamic stabilization exercises (rhythmic stabilization)
Closed kinetic chain exercises
Proprioception training
Abstain from throwing

Phase two—intermediate phase

Goals

Progress strengthening exercise
Restore muscular balance (external/internal rotation)
Enhance dynamic stability
Control flexibility and stretches

Exercises and modalities

Continue stretching and flexibility (especially internal rotation and horizontal adduction)
Progress isotonic strengthening
—Complete shoulder program
—Thrower's Ten program
Rhythmic stabilization drills
Initiate core strengthening program
Initiate leg program

Phase three—advanced strengthening phase

Goals

Aggressive strengthening
Progress neuromuscular control
Improve strength, power, and endurance
Initiate light throwing activities
Exercises and modalities
Flexibility and stretching
Rhythmic stabilization drills
Thrower's Ten program
Initiate plyometric program
Initiate endurance drills
Initiate short-distance throwing program

Phase four—return-to-activity phase

Goals

Progress to throwing program
Return to competitive throwing
Continue strengthening and flexibility drills
Exercises
Stretching and flexibility drills
Thrower's Ten program
Plyometric program
Progress interval throwing program to competitive throwing

Phase one-acute phase

The primary goals of the initial rehabilitation phase are to improve flexibility, reestablish baseline dynamic stability, normalize muscle balance, and restore proprioception without causing shoulder irritation or pain. One of the goals-to diminish the athlete's pain and inflammation -is accomplished through the use of local therapeutic modalities such as ice, ultrasound, and electrical stimulation. In addition, the athlete's activities (such as throwing and exercises) must be modified to a pain-free level.

The thrower is often instructed to abstain from throwing until advised by the physician or rehabilitation specialist. Additionally, active-assisted motion exercises have been shown to assist in reducing the athlete's pain. Another essential goal during the first phase of rehabilitation is to normalize shoulder motion, particularly shoulder internal rotation and horizontal adduction. It is common for the overhead thrower to exhibit a significant loss of internal rotation. This may be due to soft tissue tightness, which may be from muscle inflexibility due to significant and repetitive eccentric muscle forces during arm deceleration. If the posterior soft tissue structures such as the infraspinatus and teres minor muscles are tight, increased anterior translation of the humeral head may result. Therefore, the thrower should perform specific stretches and flexibility exercises for the benefit of the posterior rotator cuff muscles.

The loss of internal rotation is due to osseous adaptation of the humerus and posterior muscle tightness. The loss of internal rotation is routinely due to posterior capsular tightness. It appears that most throwers exhibit significant posterior laxity when evaluated.

The rehabilitation specialist, in addition to helping restore glenohumeral motion, should assess the resting position and mobility of the scapula. Frequently, seen overhead throwers who exhibit a posture of rounded shoulders and a forward head. This posture may lead to muscle weakness of the scapular retractor muscles due to prolonged elongation or sustained stretches. In addition, the scapula may often appear protracted and anteriorly tilted. An anteriorly tilted scapula has been shown to contribute to subacromial impingement.

In overhead throwers, this scapular position abnormality correlate to pectoralis minor muscle tightness and lower trapezius muscle weakness. Tightness of the pectoralis minor muscle can lead to axillary artery occlusion and neurovascular symptoms such as arm fatigue, pain, tenderness, and cyanosis. The lower trapezius muscle is an important muscle in arm deceleration in that it controls scapular elevation and protraction. Weakness of the lower trapezius muscle may result in improper mechanics or shoulder symptoms.

Table 3
Principles of rehabilitation in the thrower

1. Never overstress healing tissue
2. Prevent negative effects of immobilization
3. Emphasize external rotation muscular strength
4. Establish muscular balance
5. Emphasize scapular muscle strength
6. Improve posterior shoulder flexibility
7. Enhance proprioception and neuromuscular control
8. Establish biomechanically efficient throwing
9. Gradually return to throwing activities
10. Use established criteria to progress specialist should carefully assess the position, mobility, and strength of the overhead thrower's scapula.

Throwers stretch their pectoralis minor muscle and strengthen the lower trapezius muscle and scapular retractor and protractor muscles. Additional primary goals of this first phase are to restore muscle strength, reestablish baseline dynamic stability, and restore proprioception. In this early phase of rehabilitation, the goal is to reestablish muscle balance. Therefore, the focus is on improving the strength of the weak muscles such as the external rotator muscles, the supraspinatus muscle, and the scapular muscles.

The scapular muscles routinely focus on in rehabilitation are the trapezius, serratus anterior, and rhomboid muscles. If the injured athlete is extremely sore or painful, submaximal isometric exercises should be employed; conversely, if the athlete exhibits minimal soreness, then lightweight isotonic exercises may be safely initiated.

Additionally, during this phase use rehabilitation exercise drills that are designed to restore the neurosensory properties of the shoulder capsule that has experienced microtrauma and to enhance the sensitivity of the afferent mechanoreceptors. Specific drills that restore neuromuscular control during this initial phase are rhythmic stabilization and reciprocal isometric muscle contractions for the internal/external rotator muscles of the shoulders.

Additionally, proprioceptive neuromuscular facilitation patterns are used with rhythmic stabilization and slow reversal hold to reestablish proprioception and dynamic stabilization. The purpose of these exercise drills is to facilitate agonist/antagonist muscle cocontractions. Efficient coactivation assists in restoring the balance in the force couples of the shoulder joint, thus enhancing joint congruency and joint compression.

Other exercise drills commonly used during this first rehabilitation phase include joint repositioning tasks and axial loading exercises (such as closed kinetic chain). Active joint compression stimulates the articular receptors. Thus, axial loading exercise drills such as weight shifts, weight shifting on a ball, wall pushups, and quadruped positioning drills are beneficial in restoring proprioception.

Phase two-intermcdiate phase

In phase two of the rehabilitation program, the primary goals are to progress the strengthening program, continue to improve flexibility, and facilitate neuromuscular control. During this phase, the rehabilitation program is progressed to more aggressive isotonic strengthening activities with emphasis on the restoration of muscle balance. Selective muscle activation is also used to restore muscle balance and symmetry. In the overhead thrower, the shoulder external rotator muscles, scapular retractor muscles, and protractor and depressor muscles are frequently isolated because of weakness. A core exercise program for the overhead thrower that specifically addresses the vital muscles involved in the throwing motion. This exercise program was developed on the basis of the collective EMG research of numerous investigators, and is referred to as the "Thrower's Ten Program ."

Sidelying external rotation and prone rowing into external rotation have been shown to elicit the highest amount of EMG activity of the posterior rotator cuff muscles. The scapula provides proximal stability to the shoulder joint, enabling distal segment mobility. Scapular stability is vital for normal asymptomatic arm function. Several authors have emphasized the importance of scapular muscle strength and neuromuscular control in contributing to normal shoulder function.Isotonic exercise techniques are used to strengthen the scapular muscles. Furthermore, Wilk also developed specific exercise drills to enhance neuromuscular control of the scapulothoracic joint. These exercise drills are designed to maximally challenge the scapulothoracic muscle force couples and to stimulate the proprioceptive and kinesthetic awareness of the scapula. Another popular exercise used by athletes is the "empty can" exercise. With this exercise movement, the arm is placed in the scapular plane with the hand placed in full internal rotation (thumb down).

Recently, several investigators have tested the efficiency of this exercise. Furthermore, the investigators noted that the empty can exercise produced high EMG activity but only when the arm was elevated from 90° to

120°, which places the upper extremity into an impingement type of position. Many times when athletes perform the empty can exercise they complain of shoulder pain during this maneuver. The shoulder pain may be occurring because of superior displacement of the humeral head due to weakness of the external rotator muscles.

Overhead throwing athletes often exhibit external rotator muscle weakness; thus, advocate the "full can" exercise instead of the empty can exercise in an attempt to avoid the possibility of causing superior humeral head displacement, which may lead to pain and inflammation. Also during this second rehabilitation phase, the overhead throwing athlete is instructed to perform core.

Phase three-advanced strengthening phase

In phase three, the advanced strengthening phase, the goals are to initiate aggressive strengthening drills, enhance power and endurance, perform functional drills, and gradually initiate throwing activities. During this phase, the athlete performs the Thrower's Ten exercise program, continues manual resistance stabilization drills, and initiates plyometric drills. Dynamic stabilization drills are also performed to enhance proprioception and neuromuscular control. These drills include rhythmic stabilization exercise drills by throwing a ball into a wall, push-ups onto a ball, and ball throws. Plyometric training may be used to enhance dynamic stability, enhance proprioception, and gradually increase the functional stresses placed on the shoulder joint. Plyometric exercise employs three phases, all intended to use the elastic and reactive properties of the muscle to generate maximum force production.

The first phase is the eccentric phase, where a rapid prestretch is applied to the musculotendinous unit, stimulating the muscle spindle. The second phase is the amortization phase, representing the time between the eccentric and concentric phases. This time should be as short as possible so that the beneficial neurologic effects of the prestretch are not lost. The final phase is the resultant concentric contraction. Wilk et al. established a plyometric exercise program for the overhead thrower. The initial plyometric program consists of two-handed exercise drills such as a chest pass, overhead soccer throw, side-to-side throws, and side throws.

The goal of the plyometric drills is the transfer of energy from the legs and trunk to the upper extremity. Once these two-handed exercise drills are mastered, the athlete is progressed to one-handed drills. These drills include standing onehanded throws in a functional throwing position, wall dribbling, and plyometric step and throws.

Additionally, muscle endurance exercises should be emphasized for the overhead thrower. Once the thrower was fatigued, shoulder external rotation decreased and ball velocity diminished, as did lead knee flexion and shoulder adduction torque. A relationship between muscle fatigue and diminished proprioception. Specific endurance exercise drills use include wall dribbling with a Plyoball (Functional Integrated Technologies, Watsonville, California), wall arm circles, upper body cycle, or isotonic exercises using lower weights with higher repetition.

Other techniques that may be beneficial to enhance endurance include throwing an underweighted or overweighted ball (that is, a ball that is either less than or more than the weight of an official baseball). These techniques are designed to enhance training, coordination, and the transfer of kinetic energy. Conversely, the overweighted ball is generally used to enhance shoulder strength and power. Also, during this third rehabilitation phase an interval throwing program may be initiated. Before initiating such a program, occasionally suggest that the athlete perform "shadow" throwing or mirror throwing, which is the action of mimicking the throwing mechanics into a mirror, but not actively throwing. This is designed to allow the athlete to work on proper throwing mechanics before throwing a baseball. The interval throwing program is initiated once the athlete can fulfill these specific criteria:

1) satisfactory clinical examination,
2) nonpainful range of motion,
3) satisfactory isokinetic test results, and
4) appropriate rehabilitation progress.

The interval throwing program is designed to gradually increase the quantity, distance, intensity, and type of throws needed to facilitate the gradual restoration of normal biomechanics. Interval throwing is organized into two phases: phase I is a long-toss program (from 45 to 180 feet) and phase II is an off-the-mound program for pitchersa. During this third rehabilitation phase, usually initiate phase I of the interval throwing program at 45 feet and progress to throwing from 60 feet. The athlete is instructed to use a crow-hop type of throwing mechanism and lob the ball with an arc for the prescribed distance. Flat ground, longtoss throwing is used before throwing off the mound to allow the athlete to gradually increase the applied loads to the shoulder while using proper throwing mechanics. In addition, during this phase of rehabilitation, routinely allow the position player to initiate a progressive batting program. We routinely use a program that progresses the athlete from swinging a light bat, to hitting a ball off a tee, to soft-toss hitting, to batting practice.

Phase four-return-to-throwing phase

Phase four of the rehabilitation program, the return-to throwing phase, usually involves the progression of the interval throwing program. For pitchers, progress the long-toss program to 120 or 145 feet, whereas position players would progress to throwing from 180 feet. Once the pitcher has successfully completed throwing from 120 or 145 feet, the athlete is instructed to throw 60 feet from the windup on level ground. Once this step is successfully completed, phase II, throwing from the mound, is performed. Position players continue to progress the long-toss program to 180 feet, then perform fielding drills from their specific position. While the athlete is performing the interval throwing program, the clinician should carefully monitor the thrower's mechanics and throwing intensity.

In a study conducted at our biomechanics laboratory, objectively measured the throwing intensity of healthy pitchers. When pitchers were asked to throw at 50% effort, radar gun analysis indicated that the actual effort was approximately 83% of their maximum speed. When asked to throw at 75% effort, the pitchers threw at 90% of their maximum effort. This indicates that these athletes threw at greater intensities than were suggested, which may imply difficulty of controlling velocity at lower throwing intensities. In addition, during this fourth phase the thrower is instructed to continue all the exercises previously prescribed to improve upper extremity strength, power, and endurance.

The athlete is also instructed to continue the stretching program, core exercise training, and lower extremity strengthening activities. Lastly, the athlete is counseled on a year-round conditioning program based on the principles of periodization. Thus, the athlete is instructed when to begin such things as strength training and throwing. To prevent the effects of overtraining or throwing when poorly conditioned, it is critical to instruct the athlete specifically on what to do through specific exercises throughout the year. This is especially critical in preparing the athlete for the following season.

Rehabilitation Guidelines

To successfully rehabilitate the overhead thrower, an accurate differential diagnosis is imperative. Once the diagnosis is established, an appropriate rehabilitation program can be formulated.

Posterosuperior Glenoid Impingement

Posterosuperior glenoid impingement, often referred to as internal impingement, is one of the most frequently observed injuries to the overhead throwing athlete. One of the underlying causes of symptomatic internal impingement is excessive anterior shoulder laxity. One of the primary goals of the rehabilitation program is to enhance the athlete's dynamic stabilization abilities, thus controlling anterior humeral head translation. Another essential goal is to restore flexibility to the posterior rotator cuff muscles of the glenohumeral joint. Additionally, the program emphasizes muscle strengthening of the posterior rotator cuff to reestablish muscle balance and improve joint compression abilities.

The scapular muscle must be an area of increased focus as well. Restoring dynamic stabilization is an essential goal to minimize the anterior translation of the humeral head during the late cocking and early acceleration phases of throwing. Exercise drills such as proprioceptive neuromuscular facilitation patterns with rhythmic stabilization are incorporated. Also, stabilization drills performed at end-range external rotation are beneficial in enhancing dynamic stabilization.

Perturbation training of the shoulder joint is performed to enhance proprioception, dynamic stabilization, and neuromuscular control. This form of training has been extremely effective in treating the thrower who has posterior/superior impingement. Once we have restored posterior flexibility, normalized glenohumeral strength ratios, enhanced scapular muscle strength, and diminished the patient's symptoms, an interval throwing program may be initiated. Some suggested abstaining from throwing for 2 to 12 weeks before the throwing program, depending on the thrower's symptoms. Once the thrower begins the interval throwing program, the clinician or pitching coach should observe the throwing mechanics frequently. Occasionally, throwers who exhibit internal impingement will allow their arm to lag behind the scapula, thus throwing with excessive horizontal abduction and not throwing with the humerus in the plane of the scapula. Some colleagues, referred to this as "hyperangulation" of the arm. This type of fault leads to excessive strain on the anterior capsule and to internal impingement of the posterior rotator cuff.

Correction of throwing pathomechanics is critical to returning the athlete to asymptomatic and effective throwing.

Overuse syndrome tendinitis

Occasionally, throwers will describe the symptoms and exhibit the signs of overuse tendinitis of the shoulder musculature. The tendinitis signs and symptoms can be of the rotator cuff or of the long head of the biceps brachii muscles, or both. These signs frequently occur early in the season, when the athlete's arm is not in the best condition. They can also occur at the end of the competitive season when the athlete begins to fatigue. Additionally, these signs develop when the athlete does not perform the in-season strengthening program while throwing. Mere participation in throwing activities does not ensure the maintenance of proper shoulder muscle strength and flexibility. Specific muscles (external rotator muscles, scapular muscles) often become weak and painful because of the stresses involved with throwing.

The rehabilitation program for overuse rotator cuff muscle tendinitis should concentrate on treating the cause(s) of the tendinitis and not merely the symptoms. The athlete is often instructed to discontinue throwing for a short period (2 to 4 weeks) to reduce inflammation and restore strength and flexibility. Other times, the athlete is instructed to reduce the number of throws during competition or practice. Thus, a strict pitch count is enforced. The rehabilitation program will be successful if the cause is identified, throwing activities are modified, and proper strength and flexibility are restored. Often, the thrower will complain of bicipital pain, occasionally referred to as "groove pain." The biceps brachii muscle appears to be moderately active during the overhead throwing motion. Bicipital tendinitis that is present in the overhead thrower usually represents a secondary condition. The primary disorder may be instability, a SLAP (superior labral, anterior and posterior) lesion, or some similar malady. The rehabilitation of this condition focuses on improving dynamic stabilization of the glenohumeral joint through muscle training drills.

The stimulation of the anterior capsule caused a reflexive biceps muscle contraction. They demonstrated that the biceps brachii muscle was the first muscle to reflexively respond to stimulation of the capsule, occurring in 2.7 msec. Therefore, it is the belief of one of the authors (KEW) that the biceps brachii muscle is activated to a greater extent when the thrower exhibits hyperlaxity or inflammation of the capsule. Furthermore, higher EMG activity in amateur throwers compared with skilled throwers. Nonoperative rehabilitation for this condition usually consists of a reduction in throwing activities and reestablishment of dynamic stability and modalities such as ice, ultrasound, iontophorosis, and electrical stimulation to reduce bicipital inflammation.

Posterior rotator cuff musculature tendinitis

The successful treatment of posterior rotator cuff musculature tendinitis, or tensile rotator cuff musculature failure, depends on its differential diagnosis from internal impingement. Frequently, the athlete complains of pain in the same location for both lesions. However, subjectively the athlete notes posterior shoulder pain during the deceleration phase of throwing. Conversely, athletes who exhibit internal impingement complain of pain during the late cocking and early acceleration phases. During the deceleration phase of the overhead pitch, the distraction forces at the glenohumeral joint approach one to one and a half times body weight. These are excessive forces that must be dissipated and opposed by the posterior rotator cuff muscles. Pitchers occasionally exhibit this condition. Once the athlete is examined, the most common findings are significant posterior rotator cuff muscle weakness, weakness of the lower trapezius muscle and scapular retractor muscles, and tightness of the posterior rotator cuff muscles. The rehabilitation program focuses on several key areas. First, throwing activities are discontinued until the athlete exhibits proper muscle strength ratios between the external and internal rotator muscles. This ratio should be at least 64% (optimal goal, 66% to 75%). Second, the athlete is placed on an aggressive strengthening program for the posterior rotator cuff muscles and the retractor and depressor muscles of the scapula. Exercises that emphasize are sidelying external rotation, prone rowing into external rotation, prone horizontal abduction with external rotation, scapular retraction, and prone horizontal abduction.

Once strength levels have improved, the exercise program should emphasize eccentric muscle training. In particular, the external rotator muscles and the lower trapezius muscle are the focus of the eccentric program. The EMG activity of the teres minor muscle is 84% and that of the lower trapezius muscle is 78% of a maximum voluntary isometric contraction during the deceleration phase of the throw. These two muscles are the most active during this phase and, thus, must be the focus of the strengthening program. In addition, flexibility and stretching exercises for the posterior rotator cuff muscles are performed throughout the rehabilitation program. Also use heat and ultrasound before stretching to enhance tissue extensibility while increasing circulation to the area. Once flexibility and muscle strength are improved and the athlete's pain and inflammation have abated, an interval throwing program can be initiated. The interval throwing program should be progressed slowly so that the stresses of throwing are gradually increased. The athlete is instructed to be sure to follow through properly and not to terminate the deceleration phase abruptly, which may lead to increased stresses on the posterior rotator cuff muscles.

SLAP Lesions

The nonoperative treatment of SLAP lesions depends on the type of lesion present. Throwers who exhibit this type of lesion are treated with a program similar to the posterosuperior glenoid impingement protocol. Conversely, players with a type II or type IV SLAP lesion are probably best served by undergoing surgical intervention. If rehabilitation is indicated before surgery, the program should emphasize restoration of range of motion through stretching exercises within the patient's tolerance. Avoidance of overhead motions with excessive internal/external rotation is enforced because of possible joint snapping and pain. A strengthening program should be performed in an attempt to prevent muscle atrophy. The strengthening exercises should be performed with the arm below shoulder level to prevent further damage to the glenoid labrum.

Strengthening exercises such as external/internal rotation with the arm at the side or scapular plane, scapular strengthening, and deltoid muscle exercises to 90° of abduction can be safely performed. Exercises such as shoulder press, bench press, and latissimus dorsi muscle pulldowns (behind the neck) are avoided because of increased stress applied to the superior labrum and anterior glenohumeral glenohumeral joint capsule. Furthermore, the clinician should be cautious with closed kinetic chain exercises that result in excessively high joint compressive loads that could result in further compromise of the glenoid labrum.

Subacromial impingement

Primary subacromial impingement in the young professional baseball player is unusual, but it may occur. Subacromial impingement complaints in this group of athletes usually represent primary hyperlaxity leading to secondary impingement. In cases of abnormal acromial architecture, the athlete may require surgical treatment. The nonoperative treatment for subacromial impingement should focus on a five-step program. First, abstain from irritating activities such as throwing or other overhead motions for 7 to 10 days, until inflammation is diminished. Second, normalize glenohumeral motion and capsular mobility. The patients with inferior capsular tightness frequently complain of subacromial pain. Thus, the rehabilitation program must focus on restoring normal capsular and soft tissue mobility posteriorly and inferiorly.

The third step is to enhance dynamic stability of the glenohumeral and scapulothoracic joint. Thus, the rehabilitation program must focus on rotator cuff muscle strength to adequately compress and stabilize the humeral head within the glenoid fossa. Furthermore, scapular strengthening should also be an area of focus. During arm elevation, the scapula upwardly rotates, retracts, and posteriorly tilts. Some reported that patients with impingement exhibit less posterior tilting than do subjects without impingement. Thus, the rehabilitation program should include pectoralis minor muscle stretching and inferior trapezius muscle strengthening to ensure posterior scapular tilting. This is especially true with the recreational baseball player who performs a sedentary job. The fourth step is to emphasize the retractor muscles of the scapula and to correct any forward-head posture. Thus, employ scapular retractionstrengthening exercises. The last step is a gradual return to throwing activities once pain has significantly diminished.

The successful nonoperative treatment of throwing athletes with ossification of the posterior capsule is often difficult. It has been our clinical experience that the thrower with symptomatic thrower's exostosis can be conservatively managed for some time; however, long-term success is limited and often surgical debridement of the ossification may become necessary. Nonoperative treatment includes abstaining from throwing until pain subsides, restoring posterior capsule and muscle flexibility, improving posterior rotator cuff musculature and scapular strength, and a gradual return to throwing activities.

Primary Instability

Most skillful throwers exhibit significant hyperelasticity of their anterior glenohumeral joint capsule, which allows excessive external rotation and proper throwing mechanics. Because of the repetitive microtraumatic forces of throwing, the hyperelasticity may progress to primary instability and associated lesions and complaints. This is a very common occurrence in the overhead thrower.

The key aspects are reduction of throwing activity to allow diminished inflammation, normalization of motion, restoration of proper strength of glenohumeral and scapular muscles, enhancement of proprioception, and a gradual return to throwing. In the majority of cases, this treatment will be effective.

Acute traumatic instability

An acute traumatic dislocation to a throwing athlete's dominant shoulder can be devastating. The injury may include a Bankart lesion, rotator cuff muscle tear, labral tear, or even injury to the brachial plexus muscle. The treatment for a dislocation in the thrower is surgical correction. Before surgery, the athlete's shoulder should be placed in a sling for comfort. In addition, gentle range of motion exercises should be performed to gradually restore motion before surgery. A mild strengthening program for the glenohumeral and scapular muscles should also be performed with the goal of preventing muscle atrophy and weakness and loss of dynamic stabilization.

Improper mechanics

Throwing with improper or faulty mechanics can lead to shoulder pain or injury, or both, because of the abnormal stresses that are applied across various tissues. To determine whether the thrower exhibits improper throwing mechanics, the clinician should carefully observe the athlete throw. Obvious flaws can be seen occasionally. The clinician may often require assistance from an experienced and knowledgeable baseball coach. The skilled eye of an experienced coach can frequently determine subtle abnormalities in the throwing mechanics. Perhaps the most objective analysis is a high-speed video biomechanical evaluation. This can be done at a biomechanics laboratory using specialized high-speed video cameras and computer analysis of the data. When evaluating an athlete's throwing mechanics, commonly look at several different aspects of the movement. The clinician can use a video recorder to film the thrower and analyze the biomechanics during slow-motion playback to pinpoint improper mechanics. Filming should be performed from multiple views to accurately assess the athlete, including lateral (facing the athlete), posterior, and anterior views. There are several aspects of the throwing motion in sequential order to detect subtle pathomechanical deviations through the phases of throwing. Biomechanical analysis of the throwing motion begins with the lateral view; there are several critical moments to observe from this view.

During the wind-up phase, the pitcher should be in a balanced position when the lead leg reaches the highest point. Forward movement should not begin until the lead leg is fully raised. Rushing the delivery by falling toward home plate during the wind-up phase may decrease the amount of energy generated by the lower body and result in a loss of velocity. As the athlete begins the early cocking phase, the path of motion as the thrower removes the ball from the glove should be smooth, with the elbow flexed and the fingers on top of the ball. As the lead leg comes in contact with the ground, the knee should be slightly flexed and the elbow should be level with the shoulder. A right-handed pitcher will show the ball to the shortstop and a left-handed pitcher will show the ball to the second baseman. The stride should be long enough to allow sufficient rotation and force generation from the hips and trunk, approximately equal to the height of the thrower. At maximal external rotation during the late cocking phase, the arm should be abducted approximately 90° to 100°.

Some reported that throwing with reduced external rotation at the time of foot contact causes an increase in strain on the shoulder during acceleration and ball release. Furthermore, the thrower should begin straightening the elbow before shoulder internal rotation during the acceleration phase. At this time, the lead leg extends, or straightens, to stabilize the body and provide a fulcrum for body rotation. During the deceleration and follow-through phases, the throwing shoulder should internally rotate and horizontally adduct across the body. The upper extremity should cross the front of the body and end outside the lead leg. Abbreviating the follow-through and ending with the hand toward the target may increase the stresses applied to the shoulder. Observing the thrower from a posterior view allows the clinician to observe two instants during the throwing motion. As the thrower removes the ball from the glove during early cocking, the arm path should move smoothly in a down, back, and upward motion as the thrower strides toward the target.

A thrower whose arm moves behind the body may cause excessive anterior capsular straining and possible internal impingement. Also of interest from the posterior view is the hand position during late cocking. As previously stated, the ball should be facing the shortstop for right-handed throwers and the second baseman for left-handed throwers. An anterior view of the throwing motion is helpful to the clinician to determine the position of the stride leg as the foot comes into contact with the ground. At this time, the lead foot should be pointed toward the target. Often young and inexperienced throwers overrotate and place the lead foot on the first base side of the mound.

This results in the pitcher's "opening up too soon" and causes the hips to rotate early, resulting in loss of velocity and increased strain to the anterior shoulder.

Some shown that as the lead foot angle becomes more open, the thrower tends to throw across the body and increases the loads applied to the shoulder. Furthermore, "leading with the elbow" (increased horizontal adduction and elbow flexion) during the acceleration phase correlated to decreased loads at the shoulder but increased loads on the medial aspect of the elbow. The orientation of the shoulder at the moment of ball release can also be assessed from the anterior view of the throwing motion. The throwing elbow should be in line with the shoulder with minimal flexion of the elbow. The nonthrowing elbow should be tucked at the side. As the athlete progresses into the deceleration and followthrough phases, the throwing arm should follow a long arc of deceleration, allowing proper dissipation of forces from the arm to the trunk and lower extremities.

Overhead throwing athletes typically have a unique musculoskeletal profile. The overhead thrower frequently experiences shoulder pain because of anterior capsular laxity and increased demands placed on the dynamic stabilizers. This may be the result of repetitive high stresses imparted to the shoulder joint and may lead to the development of injuries.

Most commonly, these injuries are overuse injuries and can be successfully managed with a well-structured rehabilitation program. The rehabilitation program should focus on the correction of adaptive changes seen in the overhead thrower, such as loss of internal rotation and muscle weakness of the external rotator muscles and scapular muscles. The rehabilitation specialist may then initiate the athlete's gradual throwing program to return to competition.

The athlete's overhead throwing motion should be examined to determine whether improper biomechanics are contributing to the injury. Lastly, education of the athlete in the area of year-round conditioning is imperative. The overhead throwing athlete should be instructed as to when to begin conditioning and throwing to prepare for the next competitive season and prevent subsequent injury.

3

Female Softball Athlete

The relationship between proprioception and injury remains unclear. It is unknown whether shoulder "overuse" injuries suffered by athletes who perform overhand motions result from altered proprioception that is caused by the nature of the sport, or if the injuries cause a decrease in proprioception, leading to further damage. This lack of clarity has prompted researchers to evaluate proprioception in the shoulder of the throwing athlete.

The two most common methods of measuring shoulder joint proprioception include threshold to detection of passive movement and joint position sense. Threshold to detection of passive movement can be measured with a proprioception testing device or an isokinetic dynamometer. Typically, these devices measure rotational angle and generate a specific velocity of movement for the joint being tested. Starting with the subject's limb at a predetermined angle, researchers ask subjects to indicate when they first detect movement.

The device typically surrounds the subject's arm and provides tactile feedback to the subject throughout the maneuver. The subject also must interpret the movement in one limb and activate a trigger switch with the other to identify their threshold. This measurement situation could result in errors because of the coordination needed between limbs. Some researchers have attempted to limit the amount of tactile feedback from the device by using specialized pneumatic cuffs to provide joint motion. It is possible, however, that this method provides more tactile feedback than when the limb is unattached and free to move in space. For example, prophylactic taping and bracing have been shown to improve proprioception in the ankle and knee.

The prophylactic treatment may augment afferent input by providing increased cutaneous stimulation. Joint position sense can be assessed by active reproduction of passive positioning of a limb. The limb is passively moved to a predetermined angle and held for a few seconds. The subject relaxes and returns the limb to the starting position. The subject then attempts to actively reposition the limb to the target angle.

The difference between the target angle and the repositioned angle is then calculated and used for statistical analysis. Increases in threshold to detection of passive movement have been demonstrated in both internal and external rotation in pre- and postexercised shoulders. From a practical standpoint, the muscles of the overhand throwing athlete may fatigue during competition, and this could decrease the threshold, which could ultimately affect performance and predispose the athlete to injury. Joint position sense has also been shown to decrease after fatigue. In one study, the target angles were chosen near the end-range of motion. It was originally thought that, because the capsule was tighter at the end of the range, this position provided most of the information for joint position sense. However, because joint position sense was decreased after fatigue, the authors suggested that the rotator cuff plays a large role in shoulder proprioception. Others have also suggested that joint position sense is more accurately assessed near the end-range of motion, where there is greater tension on the restraints to movement. All of these studies have combined male and female subjects or evaluated male subjects only. There is a paucity of research on joint position sense in female athletes, particularly female overhand athletes.

One of the few studies involving female softball players examined muscle firing patterns in the shoulder region. Some researche study suggested that the muscle-firing pattern in the shoulder of female fast-pitch softball players is not significantly different from that in overhand baseball pitchers. Their findings may imply that the injuries characteristic in female softball athletes may be similar to those in male throwing athletes.

The shoulder injuries are common in women's softball, and that significant time loss during the season can result from injuries to the throwing arm of pitchers. Thus, further study into potential causes of injury in the female athlete involved in overhand throwing sports and, more specifically, the softball athlete, is needed. Hypothesized that there would be an increase in external rotation joint position sense scores in the dominant shoulder of the softball athlete as compared with scores in the nondominant shoulder and as compared with scores in both shoulders of the female nonthrowing athlete.

Instrumentation

Range of motion and joint position sense were measured by using an inclinometer. The inclinometer is a flat goniometer with 360 individual markings inscribed as single degrees around the circumference. The needle on the inside of the inclinometer is compared with the degree markings on the outside to determine the angle measured. The needle is fixed to the center of the inclinometer and is allowed to rotate freely inside. Because it can move without any restrictions, gravity maintains the needle in a downward position. When the limb is moved, the needle remains in this position, allowing for the angle measurement. Intratester and intertester reliabilities were established before data collection began (intraclass correlation coefficient [ICC] 2,1 0.99 and 0.99, respectively).

The inclinometer was attached to the arm of a Kin-Com dynamometer, and two researchers recorded measurements of 10 different angles repeated three times each. The three trials derived from each of the 10 different angles by the primary investigator (GCD) were compared to determine intratester reliability, whereas the first measurement taken by both testers at each of these different angles was compared to determine intertester reliability.

Table 1

Subject Demographic Data (Mean SD)

Group	*Age (years)*	*Height (cm)*	*Mass (kg)*
Softball (N=50)	19.0± 0.9	166.9± 6.1	68.2±11.9
Nonthrowing (N=50)	19.3 ± 1.3	167.5 ± 7.2	61.7±6.5
Total	19.2±1.2	167.2±6.6	64.9±10.1

Testing procedures

All testing was performed either in the Athletic Training/ Sports Medicine Research Laboratory or the respective athletic training rooms of the teams participating in the study. Subjects reported for testing on one occasion. Arm dominance was determined by asking the athletes which arm they used to throw a ball. Demographic information was then recorded for all subjects. Each athlete's dominant and nondominant active shoulder range of motion was determined for internal and external rotation, flexion, and extension at the beginning of the test session. The inclinometer was secured on the lateral side of the subject's wrist with a VELCRO strap just proximal to the ulnar styloid process for the internal and external rotation testing and just proximal to the elbow joint for the flexion and extension measurements.

A coin toss was used to determine which sets of movements (internal/ external rotation versus flexion/ extension) were performed first. A second coin toss was then performed to determine which specific movement (internal versus external rotation or flexion versus extension) was measured first within these sets. During the active range of motion exercise and joint repositioning, the subject was instructed to make a fist with the involved hand to decrease any extraneous movement at the hand and wrist.

Active range of motion for internal and external rotation was measured with the subject in the supine position with the shoulder abducted and the elbow flexed to 90°. The internal and external rotation testing was performed with the subject supine so that the scapula was stabilized by the table, thereby reducing scapular substitution. In an effort to reduce tactile feedback to the subjects, we did not use any other device or restraint to further stabilize the trunk or the scapula. The flexion and extension movements were measured with the subject standing. While in this position, the subject was instructed to maintain an upright posture and to avoid arching her back. If the subject moved the trunk during any of the range of motion or joint position sense measurements, the trial was repeated. Again, no restraints were used during the flexion and extension measurements. The subjects to keep the forearm in a single plane during all range of motion and joint position sense testing. The subjects reported no difficulty in following these instructions and only a few tests had to be repeated. Immediately after these measurements were taken, a blindfold was applied and the joint position sense testing began.

Joint position sense testing first required a calculation of the target angle based on the range of motion measurements. The target angle by subtracting 10% of the total range of motion (external rotation internal rotation or flexion extension) from the specific range of motion being tested. Percentage of the total range of motion so that each subject would experience the same relative target angle. A sample calculation for external and internal rotation target angles is as follows: external rotation range of motion = 100°, internal rotation range of motion = 80°; thus, the total range of motion + external + internal rotation = 180°. To determine the target angle for external rotation, take 10% of 180° = 18°; therefore, 100° - 18° = 82° will be the target angle for external rotation for this subject. Likewise, for internal rotation, 80° - 18° = 62°; thus, 62° would be the target angle for internal rotation for this subject.

Target angles for all four movements in both the dominant and nondominant shoulders were calculated.

These target angles were then used for the subject to aim for during the repositioning required for the joint position sense testing. Specifically, moved the subject's limb to the target angle and held it in place for 3 seconds. The subject was then told to relax and actively return the arm to the neutral starting position. During the internal/external rotation testing, the neutral position was achieved when the forearm was perpendicular to the table (0° of shoulder rotation).

During the flexion/extension testing, the neutral position was achieved when the subject's arm was relaxed at her side. Each subject was then instructed to actively return her arm to the target angle and to inform the investigator when she felt she had reproduced the original target angle. The arm was held motionless while the angle measurement was recorded. The repositioning was repeated three times for each of the four movements. Both the dominant and nondominant arms were tested. Error scores from the three repositioning trials of each movement were calculated as the difference between the repositioning trial angle and the target angle. The absolute value of this difference was averaged over the three trials and used in the statistical analysis.

A 2 × 2 × 4 mixed design analysis of variance with repeated measures on the dependent variable (error scores) was used for data analysis. The independent variables were group, arm, and movement. The between-subject variable was group status, either nonthrowing group (soccer and track athletes) or softball group. The two within-subject variables were arm (dominant and nondominant) and movements (internal and external rotation, flexion and extension). The Tukey honestly significant difference post hoc test was used to examine differences of interest. An a priori alpha level of P = 0.05 was set for all comparisons. The Statistical Package for the Social Sciences Version 10.0.0 was used for all statistical calculations. Additionally, individual range of motion measurements were compared by using dependent sample t-tests to determine whether significant differences existed between shoulders within both groups of subjects.

Range of motion

Additionally, comparisons between the dominant and nondominant shoulders are shown. In the softball group, there was significantly greater external rotation range of motion in the dominant shoulder as compared with the nondominant shoulder. Additionally, there was significantly less internal rotation range of motion in the dominant shoulder compared with the nondominant shoulder. The nonthrowing group also had significantly greater external rotation range of motion in the dominant shoulder compared with the nondominant shoulder.

Joint Position Sense

There were no differences in joint position sense error scores between pitcher and player positions in the softball group. Thus, combined all the players in the softball group for analysis. The analysis of variance revealed a significant group by movement interaction, which was demonstrated by the significantly greater external rotation error scores in the softball group compared with the external rotation error scores in the nonthrowing group.

The softball group also had greater external rotation error scores compared with their own extension error scores. The Tukey post hoc analysis determined that the difference between means needed to be 1.42° or greater to be considered statistically significant. Additionally, there was a significant movement main effect. The external rotation error score was significantly higher than the extension error score collapsed across both shoulders and groups. Interestingly, there was no group by arm interaction, despite the large external rotation mean error score in the dominant shoulder of the softball group.

Table 2

Internal and External Range of Motion Measurements.

Group and position	*Dominant*	*Nondominant*	*P value*
Softball			
Internal rotation	94.9 ± 12.8	101.9+12.6	0.000
External rotation	104.8±12.7	100.1+11.8	0.008
Nonthrowing			
Internal rotation	92.1+10.2	91.5+8.9	0.608
External rotation	97.5+11.4	93.8+12.2	0.014

Throwing athletes transfer energy from their trunk to a more injury-prone extremity during athletic competition. These athletes generally require a greater external rotation range of motion to achieve velocities necessary for the performance of their skill. Additionally, a significant difference was observed when comparing external rotation and extension joint position sense within the softball group. These findings suggest that, regardless of arm (dominant versus nondominant), external rotation joint position sense is reduced in the overhand throwing athlete. Because there is a lack of consistency across studies examining proprioception in the shoulder region, it is unclear if proprioception is affected in the dominant shoulder or both shoulders of the throwing athlete as compared with the nonthrowing athlete.

A comparison with the nondominant shoulder is typically made when clinical decisions regarding treatment and rehabilitation are performed. The relationship between proprioception and injury is unclear and is best illustrated by a paradigm presented by Lephart et al. in 1997 (Fig. 1). This paradigm shows a cycle of events involving injury, proprioceptive deficits, and instability, with no clear beginning. What makes the results from these studies interesting is the fact that, in all of them, the subjects were asymptomatic throwing athletes who had laxity occurring concomitantly with altered joint position sense. It is possible that a linear relationship exists between these factors, with laxity and reduced joint position sense occurring initially, leading to injury and the cascading cycle of events that are illustrated in the previously mentioned functional stability paradigm. However, to get a clearer understanding of these relationships, further study is warranted.

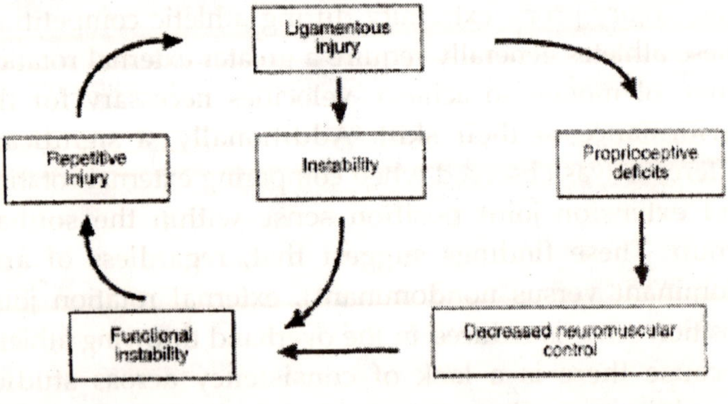

Fig. 1

Functional stability paradigm

The prefatigued error scores from that study in the dominant and nondominant shoulders were 3.3° ± 1.2° and 4.6°±1.2°, respectively, and compare favorably with the error scores calculated in the study. Rogol et al. reported slightly higher joint position sense error scores of between 5.27°±1.86° and 6.71°±3.09° in the dominant shoulder before exercise. Lephart and Fu, in a study also involving active repositioning, presented joint position sense error scores ranging from 3.0° to 5.0°. These three studies all involved male subjects.

Researchers may experience difficulty when measuring joint position sense because a number of extraneous variables may interfere with the precision of measurement. Extraneous variables can involve any feedback that is not included in the afferent information pathway from the joint and muscle receptors of the shoulder being measured. For example, visual and auditory cues are commonly controlled for during joint position testing by blindfolding the subject and playing music or white noise. In many studies that have measured proprioception, the subject is secured into a chair or fastened into a device that measures arm movement. It is possible that the increase in tactile feedback and the subject's awareness of body position while seated or lying down could account for the subtle differences in the error scores between studies.

Another factor considered was that the shoulder joint moves in all three cardinal planes. Thus, we believed it important to measure proprioception during more than just one motion. Assessing proprioception, measurements have been limited to one or two motions in one plane, most commonly internal rotation and external rotation. The addition of the flexion and extension joint position sense scores provides more information about overall shoulder joint proprioception. Each movement stresses the capsule and glenohumeral muscles differently, which could alter afferent information and affect joint position scores. Scores on two movements alone may not provide enough information about the joint position sense of the shoulder, especially considering that the external rotation joint position sense error scores have the most variability. In this study, the flexion and extension measurements were performed with the athlete standing, which may be more conducive to the athlete's ability to sense joint position. Athletes compete while standing or in the erect position and, therefore, it seems more logical to measure proprioception with the subject in that position. The position of the target angle and its relation to total range of motion may play a role in proprioception testing. A study measuring threshold to detection of passive movement in athletes participating in upper extremity sports suggested that kinesthesia was significantly improved at an angle near the end-range of motion.1 Similar findings have been reported by others.

We chose to use 90% of the full range of motion so that all subjects would have the same relative target angle as well as an angle associated with the least amount of error. It is possible that the afferent signals or proprioceptive feedback from the surrounding muscles, ligaments, and capsule increase when they are stretched as the joint moves closer to the endrange of motion. To our knowledge, the type of inclinometer used in this study has not been used in any other study. However, acknowledge that there are a few limitations of the device in measuring joint position sense. To limit the amount of tactile feedback, fixed the device to the subject solely with a VELCRO strap that was smaller in width than a typical wristwatch strap. Because the inclinometer is attached only with this strap and because there are no external devices to stabilize the shoulder, the limb is free to move in any plane of movement. If the limb moved out of the sagittal plane, the inclinometer would be raised on one side and the weighted needle of the inclinometer would not lie "true." To ensure movement in the sagittal plane, instructed the subjects to maintain their arm in the proper position and demonstrate proper limb movement before and during the joint position sense measurement. In this manner, the weighted needle was kept free to move and was able to indicate the correct repositioned angle. We were equally concerned about the reliability of the measurements produced by the inclinometer, particularly because no study to date has reported reliability coefficients. In an attempt to examine the reliability of taking reproducible readings from the inclinometer, conducted a reliability analysis before data collection. Having obtained an ICC value of 0.99, were comfortable with the reliability of our joint position sense measurements.

Joint position sense measurements taken with a Biodex isokinetic dynamometer in a study by Voight et al. had an ICC value of 0.95. The upper extremity proprioception testing device used by Allegrucci et al. produced measurements that had intrarater reliability for internal rotation and external rotation of 0.98 and 0.99, respectively. Although studies have shown similar reliability measurements, the methods used in measuring proprioception vary greatly. Researchers need to address concerns about methods and threats to validity in experiments involving joint position measurements; otherwise, conclusions may be affected.

The literature is devoid of measurements of propriocep-tion, strength, range of motion, and other measures of functional performance involving female athletes in overhand throwing sports. Although range of motion measurements were not the primary focus of our study, found that external rotation was increased in the dominant shoulder of the softball group compared with the nondominant shoulder. Additionally, internal rotation in the dominant shoulder was significantly less compared with that in the nondominant shoulder in the softball athletes. The total range of motion may not be significantly different between shoulders, but it appears to have shifted in the external rotation direction. The increase in external rotation range of motion is caused by humeral retroversion. The contention that this may be the case in both female and male athletes. Interestingly, external rotation in the dominant shoulder of the nonthrowing group was significantly higher than in the nondominant shoulder. There may be increased laxity in the female glenohumeral joint capsule, thereby allowing the dominant shoulder to have more external rotation. However, one would expect this laxity to be present in the internal rotation measurement as well, but this was not the case in the study. Additional research is needed to examine these range of motion issues further. The cause of altered proprioception in the shoulders of asymptomatic throwing athletes is unclear. Previous research has indicated that athletes in overhand sports have displayed an increase in external rotation range of motion, laxity, and altered proprioception.

These alterations may be due to congenital influences or adaptive changes that occur as a result of sport-specific requirements for overhand throwing athletes. With changes to the capsular and muscular structures around the shoulder joint, Ruffini and Pacinian corpuscles may be affected, thus resulting in partial deafferentation and proprioceptive deficits. A question of interest is whether proprioception in overhand throwing athletes could be enhanced to better coordinate the contraction and stabilizing action of the rotator cuff, which in turn could lead to fewer injuries.

Some clinicians use proprioception exercises to increase neuromuscular control and facilitate the reactive characteristics of the muscle for dynamic restraint. Proprioception exercises for the purpose of injury prevention may also be useful in addressing the deficits in joint position sense among asymptomatic overhand throwing athletes. It has been suggested that open and closed chain proprioception exercises may decrease joint position sense error scores, but it is unknown if the same holds true from an injury prevention standpoint.

Proprioception is an integral part of the rehabilitation process, and it may be prudent to use it clinically in the prevention of athletic injuries. Clinicians frequently prescribe range of motion exercises and strengthening as a part of injury prevention programs (for the shoulder and other joints). With further studies on proprioception, clinicians may be able to prescribe proprioception exercises to improve joint position sense and prevent injury.

4

General Protection in Sports

Protective equipment in sport aims to avoid or minimise injury. In general, there is little controlled evidence of the effectiveness of many types of protective equipment, but many of the principles are based on extensive experience. Each sport has its own rules and regulations for participation and play, and included in the rules there is usually a section on permitted and restricted aides or devices. Some of the protective devices are considered minimum requirements to allow participation in the sport (such as a helmet for all cycling events) whilst others will be recommended but optional (e.g. mouthguards in contact sports).

Ideally, protective equipment should satisfy the following criteria:- provide adequate protection from injuries; be comfortable to wear; affordable and if appropriate carry an approval of the relevant sporting body. Specifically it should not be used as an offensive weapon, should not provide a target for opposition, and should not impair joint function, field of vision or reaction time. Technical issues include the intended life of the equipment. For example, sporting helmets should clearly indicate whether it is for single impact or multiple impacts. The helmet should not produce dangerous fragments if damaged. Any helmet should be securely fastened but allow easy removal and should not impair thermal regulation. It is obvious that any protective equipment should not increase the risk, occurrence or severity of injury through its use either to the wearer or an opponent..

Some simple common-sense approaches are better than all of the protective braces and splints currently available. Protective equipment is not a substitute for training, preparation and acclimatisation to the sporting environment. It is recommended that people competing in a sport should train on a regular basis in all of their protective equipment to become accustomed to its weight, restrictions and overall 'feel'. In this way players are not exposed to risk of injury through inappropriate use, or inexperience with the equipment that is being used for protection from injury.

Clothing

Most sports have a particular uniform or dress code. Some sports clothing is designed to minimise heat loss and the risk of hypothermia (e.g. snow-skiing, underwater diving). Other sports have clothing which has high protection qualities (e.g. fire-proof suits for motor racing). Clothing should generally be appropriate for the prevailing environmental conditions and should protect against thermal injury (either hypo or hyperthermia).

Sun protection

Sunscreens have been shown to reduce the long term development of skin cancers and should be used in combination with other barriers such as hats, long sleeve shirts and sunglasses to minimise sun exposure on the sports field. For many outdoor sports, sun and ultra-violet exposure (which may be high and unrecognised on overcast days) is high because of prolonged periods out of the shade (e.g. fielding in cricket). Reflected rays from water or snow and ice all have the potential to burn the skin and a high sun protection factor sunscreen should be applied to all exposed skin.

Taping

Taping is the use of elasticised or rigid adhesive tape to restrict excessive, or potentially harmful motion at a joint while still allowing a desired range of motion. It is most commonly used over moderate sized joints such as the ankle, thumb and wrist. Boxers may use tape over their hands and wrists before applying boxing gloves. However, the application of tape over the skin of a joint does not strengthen that joint but merely provides additional skin proprioceptive feedback, and thus an unstable joint may require a more rigid form of bracing or complete rest from the sporting field until injury recovery has been completed. The two indications for which taping is used are:

(i)Prevention-taping is used as a preventative measure for sportspeople competing in high risk activities without an underlying structural weakness (e.g. ankle taping in basketball players) and

(ii) Rehabilitation where taping is used as a protective measure for a structurally weak joint during the recovery and rehabilitation phases of injury tissue repair.

Rigid (non-elastic) tape is most often used for restricting undesired movement at a joint. However, it has been shown that the tape holds its position and provides the desired proprioceptive feedback only whilst the adhesive is dry and in firm contact with the skin. This varies between fifteen and fifty minutes depending upon the nature and intensity of the sport and the forces applied through the tape. Tape should ideally be applied to skin which has been shaved at least 12 hours beforehand to minimise skin irritation. An adhesive skin spray can be applied to assist with tape adhesion in a sweaty individual.

The principle underlying rehabilitative taping is that injured ligaments should be maintained in a shortened position to minimise risk of re-injury. For prevention, taping should aim to maintain the ligaments in an anatomically neutral position. Tape should be of an appropriate width with overlap of the preceding layer of tape. Care must be taken to ensure no creases or folds occur in the tape as this will predispose to skin irritation and blisters.

Circulation and nerve compression can be a complication of taping which is applied too tightly, whilst the tape will be ineffective if is applied too loosely. When removing tape it is best done with a pair of tape scissors and moistening the tape may make it easier to remove. With regular application the skin may become sensitised to the tape adhesive and an allergy may develop. The cost of regular application of adhesive tape becomes quite prohibitive if large amounts are required. In general taping is labour intensive and therefore more expensive that the use of splints (bracing).

Bracing (splints)

Where long term joint protection is required, braces may be more practical and inexpensive than taping. The have the advantage of being easier to apply and less painful to remove and are less likely to cause local skin irritations. The disadvantages of braces are problems with sizing and fit of the brace, movement of the brace if not a perfect fit, the additional weight of the brace, and risk of brace failure. The simplest braces are heat-retaining neoprene sleeves that are commercially available for most of the joints of the body. This type of brace helps to retain heat in an inflamed or stiff joint but offers little mechanical support across the joint. As braces become more specialised the cost, size and weight of the brace tends to increase, and the support or restriction of abnormal or unwanted movement at a joint also becomes more controlled.

Head and Neck

Helmets

The role of a helmet is to absorb the forces and decelerate the blow at the point of impact, distribute the focal impact over a larger area, withstand surface abrasion and to protect the bone and soft tissues of the head from injury.

The use of helmets, however, increases the size and mass of the head. This may result in an increase in brain injury by a number of mechanisms. Blows that would have been glancing become more solid and thus transmit increased rotational force to the brain. These forces result in shearing stresses on neurones which may result in concussion and other forms of brain injury.

Helmets should be sports-specific to be most effective. There are a number of potential risks of inappropriate helmet use in sports. An ineffective helmet may provide the wearer with a false sense of security, encouraging risk-taking and worsening the chance of injury. Poorly designed helmets may obscure peripheral vision. As helmet requirements vary greatly between sports and there are a number of variations of helmet type, the demands of an individual sport must be considered, and then an appropriate helmet configuration, shock absorbing material and outer surface should be used. Athlete preference, and protection requirements may account for some of the variations in helmet design within a sport. The use of helmets is mandatory in some sports (such as motorised sports), recommended in others (cricket), optional in some sports (rugby union) and illegal in a few (soccer).

The ideal protective headware should provide adequate protection from injuries, be light in weight, be comfortable to wear, be affordable, should not impair field of vision, and should not impair reaction time. All helmets must be securely fastened but easily removable. The helmet must not produce dangerous fragments if damaged, it must not increase the risk of cervical spine injury. These factors should be reflected in its endorsement by the relevant sporting or Standards Association approving its use in the designated sport. The helmet should clearly indicate whether it is intended for single or multiple impacts, it should not provide a target for opponents and it should never be used as an offensive weapon.

Motorsport helmets are composed of a hard outer shell (usually made of fibreglass or polypropylene) with a large amount of internal padding. This padding is full contact to ensure a snug fit of the helmet and prevent twisting of the helmet over the head. Helmets for motor sport need to withstand high velocity impacts and are thus designed as single impact use, which means they should be discarded and replaced following an accident. These type of helmets have the largest helmet weight and strong cervical muscles are required to wear a helmet such as this and withstand the high gravitational forces applied in motorsports.

There are a number of different styles of helmet but the type offering the most protection is the full-face style, which includes a low protective bar across the jaw and also provides some support to the upper cervical spine. This type of helmet contains a built-in face-shield usually of clear perspex of polycarbonate to protect the eyes and face from flying debris or insects.

Another style of helmet is the open-face type which offers little protection to the face, and the profile of the helmet is higher on the head. For his reason the open-face helmet offers no support for the upper cervical spine in the event of a crash. All motorsport helmets are securely fastened under the lower jaw with an adjustable chin-strap and are compulsory equipment. Cycling helmets are also designed to withstand a single impact and have been shown to markedly reduce the incidence of head injury in wearers.

There are four basic types of helmet classified according to their construction. They are the hard shell, racing shell, soft shell and hard shell with vents. The hard shell and racing shell have a smooth outer shell of injection moulded plastic or fibreglass and a softer inner lining. Contact with the head is primarily around the brim of the helmet so that an air-space exists between the crown of the head and the helmet lining. The smooth outer lining helps with reduction in air resistance and so these models are preferred by competitive cyclists. The soft shell and hard shell with vents have an overall similar shape to the hard shell helmet but the major construction material is the polystyrene or polypropylene inner. This type of helmet offers less protection from penetrating injuries, but is more comfortable, as it allows air to circulate and heat to be dissipated more rapidly than the hard shell helmets. For these reasons this type of helmet is preferred by recreational cyclists.

Cycling helmets are secured under the lower jaw with a chin-strap that must be correctly adjusted to ensure a snug fit. The wearing of cycling helmets is compulsory in some countries (eg. Australia) but worldwide at the current point in time the majority of bicycle commuters and recreational cyclists have no legal enforcement (eg. China). The need for head protection in cyclists, particularly children, cannot be overemphasised.

Basketball, Softball and Cricket helmets have a different type of construction and purpose. These helmets are all designed as multiple impact helmets. Their primary function is to protect the head from being struck by a ball or batting implement. In baseball and softball the use of a helmet is compulsory for the batter and for running between bases. The helmet is usually constructed of injection moulded plastic or fibreglass with a double ear-flap. This helmet is not necessarily secured under the lower jaw but fits snugly to the head via the ear protection. In cricket the helmet is optional for the batting team but often worn when batting against fast bowlers. This helmet is secured under the lower jaw and most often has an attached face-shield made of either carbon steel, aluminium or perspex. This type of helmet is also optional, but recommended, for players fielding in positions closer to the batter or batsman.

American Football helmets are compulsory for players in all positions. The helmets are composed of an outer shell of hard resilient, plastic and an inner lining of either foam pads if air filled cells. The helmet covers all of the head from the eyebrows in front, over the crow of the head to the upper neck. The helmet is completed in front by a face mask made of either aluminium, carbon steel or a resilient plastic. Additional pads anchor the helmet to the cheeks and side of the face and a chin-strap securely fastens the helmet to prevent any movement.

Ice-Hockey helmets are similar to American football helmets but have a narrower profile, flatter crown and a closer face-mask. They are also composed of a lighter plastic and have less interior padding. This makes the helmet much lighter in weight that a football helmet. Helmets with face-masks and fastened chin straps are compulsory in ice-hockey and have been demonstrated to reduce the incident of head and facial trauma. In Field-Hockey only the goal-keeper wears a helmet and this is of a similar construction to the ice-hockey helmet. These helmets are designed as multiple impact helmets but must be inspected regularly for cracks of faults at which time they must be replaced.

Protective eyewear

The majority of eye injuries occur in a small number of

sports, usually the result of bodily contact, or accidental contact with a ball, shuttlecock or implement. Many people require glasses or contact lenses for visual acuity in daily living but, may neglect to wear them on the sports field. The perfect eye protector for sport should be able to prevent ocular injury without creating other injuries or restricting the fields vision. It should be comfortable, securely mounted on the head, have a strong, preferably single-piece frame into which are securely mounted lenses (prescription if necessary) of proven impact resistance, such as polycarbonate. However, polycarbonate cannot be used for high correction prescriptions, so that in this circumstances the ideal solution is to wear corrective contact lenses with plain eye protectors for safety.

Contact lenses are not protective in any circumstances and hard contact lenses are potentially unsafe. Glass lenses in prescription glasses are similarly unsafe for there is risk of trauma to the orbit or the eye. Some open eye guards are available which have been shown in studies to offer no more protection to the eye than wearing nothing at all.

Goggles are used by swimmers to protect eyes from chemical irritation caused by chlorination of the water in pools. Although these goggles are optional they are highly recommended to minimise eye irritation. They are usually constructed of a clear or tinted plastic and contoured to the face. They are held in position by elastic straps around the head to minimise movement when diving into the pool.

Face shields

Face shields are used in conjunction with helmets in many

sports to reduce the risk of accidental injury to the face, mouth, and eye by implements, balls or body parts. The actual construction of the face shield varies between sports but essentially the function of the face shield is to provide an obstruction to deflect an object or prevent it fro striking or hitting the face. This is usually accomplished with a series or bars or grid network interlacing across the face with gaps between the bars small enough to prevent a ball getting through.

The face mask may be permanently attached to a helmet, such as is the case with American football or ice-hockey helmets, or it may be a self-contained mask which can be used as a stand alone piece of protective equipment such s those used by baseball catches or home-plate umpires. Fencing and similar sports use faceshields with a fine mesh to prevent the foil or epee from contracting the face. This type of face shield is used as a standard piece of safety equipment in these sports. The face mask is incorporated into a hood which fits over the head to hold the face shield in position. One problem with this type of face shield is that it quite markedly restricts the field of vision of the wearer but as this sport is conducted with combatants face-to-face this has minimal impact on the sport.

Ear protection

Ear protection should be worn in a number of sports with high noise, risk of trauma or injury to the ear, or as a protective barrier t prevent damage to the ear and hearing mechanism. The major types of ear protection can be divided into a number of subcategories. Ear Plugs can be worn as a barrier to prevent water entering the external ear canal in sports such as swimming and underwater diving. They are usually composed of either a paraffin wax that van be moulded to conform to the meatus of the external canal or a waterproof foam that fits the meatus.

This second type allows more sound to enter the ear but is also not as waterproof as the waxy type. Ear plugs can also be used to reduce noise entering the ear, and are often used underneath helmets in motor racing. Ear Muffs are worn to minimise the noise entering the ear in sports such as rifle or pistol shooting. They are an essential protective device in noisy sports to minimise hearing loss associated with explosions occurring at a close range to the head. Elastic tape is used by football and rugby players to hold the ears to the side of the head to prevent lacerations behind the ears.

A second benefit of taping the ears to the side of the head is a reduction in the frequency and severity of auricular haematomas which may compromise cartilage perfusion, leading to collapse of the pins - referred to colloquially as 'cauliflower ears'. The ears should be protected from extreme cold as they supplied be end-arteries and subject to frost-bite. The is particularly important in alpine sports such as skiing and mountain-climbing. Simple insulation either by a hooded jacket or ear-muffs is usually all that is necessary.

Specific ear protection caps, manufactured from a firm plastic, with a soft foam inner, are worn by competitors in the sport of wrestling. This cap is designed to prevent to minimise trauma to the ear. The caps are secured in place by three straps which join the cup for each ear across the occiput, anterior to the crown of the head, and underneath the lower jaw. The ear cups are perforated with a series of holes to allow normal hearing.

Mouthguards

In body contact sports it is highly recommended that players wear a mouthguard. Mouthguards help to absorb and dissipate forces from a direct blow, protect the oral soft tissues from laceration and give direct protection to the teeth. A properly designed and fitted mouthguard nay also protect the mandible from fracture and could protect the wearer from concussive episodes. A mouthguard should cover the occlusal surface of the upper teeth and extend almost to the upper aspect of the gums. This ensures there is a barrier between the lips, buccal mucosa and the teeth. The mouthguard should ideally extend beyond the last tooth on each side to ensure optimum fit and coverage. Ill -fitting mouthguards can cause ulceration of the soft tissues, and fail to provide the protection the wearer assumes they are obtaining. There are four basic types of mouthguards which satisfy some or all of the above criteria.

— Stock or off the shelf mouthguards are made from a rubber compound or plastic and come in a limited size. The mouthguard is retained in the mouth by clinching it between the upper and lower teeth but this type offers the least protection against concussion and dental injury.

— *Mouth*—Formed guards are composed of a firm outer shell with a softer rubber liner. These can be heated (usually by boiling) then fitted in position when warm and bitten into. This has the effect of improving the fit, contour and comfort of the guard and is better than the Stock model in its protection of teeth.

— *Custom*—Made mouthguards are manufactured by a dentist of orthodontist using an accurate plaster cast of the individuals teeth. This mouthguard is made of a resilient thermoplastic material. Because this guard is cast on an accurate plaster mould of the teeth, comfort, fit and sport-specific modifications can be made very easily and accurately.

— *Bimaxillary*—Mouthguards are manufactured to cover both the upper and lower teeth and are usually worn following a jaw fracture or similar trauma to provide additional protection. The design of this guard is to lock the jaws into a predetermined position which makes breathing and speaking more difficult than with the other typed of guard.

There is a large variation in the cost of the different types of mouthguards related to the degree of customised fit, however, the advantages of the customised mouthguards justify the additional cost. Mouthguards should be stored if a perforated plastic box to avoid build-up of mould. Before and after use they should be thoroughly cleaned with a disinfectant and rinsed.

Neck Protection

There are no proven, practical and efficacious devices for protecting the neck form musculoskeletal injury. The best protection an athlete can have is strong musculature of the neck, obtained through appropriate training and desist from participating when suffering any neck injury. Neck injuries should be carefully assessed with functional X-rays and CT or MRI scans if indicated before return to sport.

In baseball and softball a throat guard extending below the catches face-mask is a compulsory piece of protective equipment, which is designed to protect the anterior throat structures (eg. Larynx, great vessels) from injury by direct contact with (usually) the ball. In American football, a neck orthosis is available which fits underneath the shoulder pads, and extends up the sides and back of the neck, like an upturned collar, to provide a rigid support onto which the helmet sits. This orthosis is designed to minimise neck movement and unload some of the forces applied by a direct impact upon the helmet. It does not in any way protect the neck from injury, nor does it stabilise an injured neck. Protection of the neck from further injury following trauma is achieved by application of a rigid cervical collar and head and neck support but do not permit participation in sports.

The team physician

The medical care of sport teams and events is one of the most challenging in sports medicine. It requires both specific sports medicine skills, general mediccal knowledge, knwledge of the specific sport covered, communication and management skills not usually required in everyday sports medicine practice. The interface of sports medicine and organisation requires knowledge of three areas:

— administration and management, liaison with other persons/bodies involved in the same event or team

— sports medicine

— the specific sport being covered

Medical care

The medical care of a sports team is a very enjoyable yet challenging aspect of sports medicine for a variety of reasons. It provides the opportunity of practising both preventive medicine and treatment of acute and chronic injuries within the context of a team situation, both on and off the field, an educational role and the chance to learn other skills depending on the size of the off-field team.

Good all-round knowledge of general and sports medicine is required, as team members will present both with sports injuries and general medical conditions, both acute and chronic. The team physician needs to have the ability to work within and fit in the organisational structure of the team. It is important to understand that in this situation the doctor's role is one of support: to assist team members to play to the maximum of their ability at all times.

The sports medicine team

The team physician heads the sports medicine team, which may comprise a variety of paramedical professionals, such as physiotherapists, masseurs, physical trainers, podiatrists, dietitians and sports psychologists

The team physician is often in a privileged position within the general team structure. He needs to be a good communicator with all: selectors, administrators, coaches and managers, players, opposing teams physicians and the other members of the sports medicine team. Specific ethical issues arise in the context of team care, such as the early return to competition following an injury, confidentiality with other players, team management and the media. The team needs to be familiar with these issues when they arise.

Roles

The role of the team doctor is a wide ranging one. He/she holds the ultimate responsibility for the diagnosis and management of medical and injury problems within the members of the team. This includes preventive aspects such as immunisation, and specific strategies to minimise the risk of injury throughout the season. Areas of responsibility include:

—Pre-season screening of all athletes

—Establishment of preventive measures

—Injury assessment and management

—General medical management

—Nutritional aspects

—Communication with other team members

Pre-season screening

Most team sports have a discrete playing season. The pre-season screening begins at the end of the previous season. A complete review of injury and health status of each athlete in the team should be carried out immediately after the last game of the season. Appropriate treatment, including surgical procedures, should be carried out at this stage, and appropriate rehabilitation programmes instituted during the off-season.

Content

At the commencement of training for the new season a full medical assessment of all players should be carried out. This is particularly important in the case of new players to the club. This assessment should cover the following aspects:

General health

Past history of illness and medications. Special emphasis to be made on diseases such as asthma, diabetes, epilepsy and infectious diseases

Immunisation status

— *Nutritional status:* Food intake diary

— *Neuropsychometric tests*: DSST (Digit Symbol Substitution Test). This is particularly relevant for contact sports and management of concussion.

— Musculoskeletal screening

History of previous injuries, especially those that are sport related Large joints examination. Test for generalised ligamentous laxity

— *Biomechanical assessment:* This includes assessment of gait and of posture (and lumbar function)

— *Fitness testing:* This may cover

— Body weight and/or skin folds (seven sites)

— Aerobic fitness (VO2 max or shuttle run)

— Plyometric strength (vertical jump)

— Strength, flexibility and proprioception. Isokinetic muscle testing may be useful.

— Digital Symbol Substitution Test

The purpose of the pre-season screening is several fold:

— to detect any injuries or factors predisposing to injury

— to implement rehabilitation strategies to treat any existing injuries

— to establish preventive programmes, either on an individual basis or as a routine for all team members

— to develop a data base that will assist in injury prevention in future

Prevention and Management

Prevention strategies

Early in the season, or even the pre-season period is often the best time to establish educational activities for the benefit of players and other team members in several aspects of sports medicine. Areas that can be covered are:

— the role of sports medicine

— warm up and stretching routines

— the importance of early diagnosis and treatment of injuries, both acute and chronic (overuse). The R.I.C.E. regime (acronym for Rest, Ice, Compression, Elevation)

— Nutrition aspects. Role of carbohydrates, importance of fluid replacement

— Drug use and doping regulations. Consult the team doctor before taking any over-the-counter drugs

General medical management

The establishment of baseline data is important for the management of medical conditions if and when they present in the course of the season. A good general medical history is the best baseline. The team physician needs to liaise with the individual players' family doctor with regards to general medical conditions. This is particularly relevant in the case of chronic conditions such as asthma, diabetes, epilepsy and allergies.

Nutritional aspects

Nutritional requirements for high performance in sport are specific to the type of sport. The presence of a dietitian would be beneficial to establish a base line and also adequate nutritional habits and understanding of energy requirements. Iron and calcium deficiencies, the former more often in female athletes, are often encountered in elite athletes, who need to be monitored in this regard. Fluid replacement and carbohydrate loading strategies (pre-game meal in particular) should be instituted. When travelling with a team, al meal arrangements are the responsibility of the Team Doctor in regard to their content.

Communication with other team members

— *Sports medicine team:* It is the responsibility of the team physician to ensure a good working relationship with all the members of the sports medicine team (physiotherapist, physical trainer, massage therapist, dietitian, etc.). A united supportive professional team provides confidence in a good recovery strategy following injury.

— *Athletes:* A good relationship with each individual athlete is paramount. An easy and confident approach will help the team physician gain the confidence of the athletes. Confidentiality must be maintained and the players appreciate that the doctor's main concern is the welfare of the players as individuals.

— *Management:* Coaches and managers need to be informed of all relevant facts, with the consent of the individual players. In the case of injuries, particularly when they are severe, a conservative and non-alarmist attitude will help gain the respect and confidence of all involved.

Heat acclimatization

Heat acclimatization is specific to the stress imposed on the human body. For example, passive exposure to heat induces some responses, notably an improved ability to dissipate heat. In contrast, physical training in a cool-dry environment results in metabolic, biochemical, hematologic, and cardiovascular adaptations. Heat acclimatization via strenuous exercise induces responses attributed to both passive heat exposure and training in cool environments. Table 1 illustrates these relationships.

Table 1

The effects of 14 days of passive and strenuous exercise protocols in cool and hot conditions on selected physiological responses

Physiological responses	*No exercise hot conditions*	*Exercise cool conditions*	*Exercise hot conditions*
Lower core temperature at the onset of sweating	++	+	++
Increased heat loss via radiation & convection (skin blood flow)	++	++	++
Increased plasma volume	+	+	++
Decreased heart rate	O	++	++
Decreased core body temperature	++	+	++
Decreased skin temperature	+	+	+
Altered metabolic fuel utilization	O	++	++
Increased sympathetic nervous system outflow (efferent)	+	++	++
Increased oxygen consumption	O	++	++
Improved exercise economy	O	O	+
Adaptation to exercise in a cool environment	O	++	++
Adaptation to exercise in a hot environment	+	+	++

Symbols: O = minimal effect; + = moderate effect; ++ = major effect.

Complete heat acclimatization requires up to 14 days, but the systems of the body adapt to heat exposure at varying rates. The early adaptations (initial 1-5 days) involve an improved control of cardiovascular function, including expanded plasma volume, reduced heart rate, and autonomic nervous system habituation which redirects cardiac output to skin capillary beds and active muscle. Plasma volume expansion resulting from increased plasma proteins and increased sodium chloride retention, ranges from +3 to +27%, and is accompanied by a 15-25% decrease in heart rate. This reduction of cardiovascular strain reduces rating of perceived exertion, which is proportional to central cardiorespiratory stress, also decreases during the first five days of exercise-heat exposure. Plasma volume expansion is a temporary phenomenon, which decays during the 8th to 14th days of heat acclimatization, and then is replaced by a longer-lasting reduction in skin blood flow that serves to increase central blood volume. The regulation of body temperature during exercise in the heat is critical, because of the great potential for lethal hyperthermia.

Thermoregulatory adaptations (i.e., increased sweat rate, earlier onset of sweat production), coupled with cardiovascular adjustments, result in a decreased central body temperature. This response is maximized after 5 to 8 days of heat acclimatization. However, the adaptations of eccrine sweat glands are different during humid and dry heat exposures. Heat acclimatization performed in a hot-humid condition stimulates a greater sweat rate than heat acclimatization in a hot-dry environment. Also, the absolute rate of sweating influences thermoregulation. If hourly sweat rate is small (<400-600 ml), a peripheral adaptation of whole body sweat rate may not occur. Conservation of sodium chloride (NaCl) also occurs during heat acclimatization.

The NaCl losses in sweat and urine decrease during days 3-9 of heat acclimatization, resulting in an expanded extracellular fluid volume. Subsequently, NaCl losses in sweat and urine increase toward pre-acclimatization levels, once physiologic strain (i.e., cardiovascular, thermal) moderates. Francesconi and colleagues (1993) recently demonstrated that NaCl losses, during a strenuous 10-day heat acclimatization protocol, were related to plasma renin (PR) and plasma aldosterone (A) concentrations. When subjects consumed a low salt diet (4g NaCl per day) and a moderate salt diet (8g NaCl per day), both PR and A increased during the first four days of heat acclimatization, but decreased during the remaining 6 days of heat acclimatization. The improved cardiovascular stability, which occurred on days 1-4 of heat acclimatization, allowed equivalent exercise performance with both diets and apparently reduced the stimulation and need for large elevations of PR and A. No change in plasma levels of arginine vasopressin (AVP) were observed across time, in either dietary group, possibly because hourly water intake matched the fluid lost in sweat. Usually, AVP synthesis is stimulated by an increase in plasma osmolarity or alterations in blood pressure, plasma volume, and renal or hepatic blood blow.

Therefore, it is unlikely that the ability to successfully sustain exercise, during the latter days of the heat acclimatization process, is specifically related to the action of hormones that regulate fluid-electrolyte balance. This is particularly true when salt balance has been achieved. Excess dietary water and electrolytes do not speed the process of heat acclimatization. When dehydration or salt deficits exist, however, cardiovascular and thermoregulatory responses may be negatively affected, and the theoretical risk of heat illness increases. Consistent daily monitoring of body weight will allow athletes to recognize water deficits which require consumption of fluid (-2 to -

3% of body weight), reduction of training duration/ intensity (-4 to -6%), or consultation with an experienced physician (in excess of -7%). Plasma cortisol concentration generally indicates the strain experienced by the body. Heat-acclimated, well-hydrated humans exhibit no change in plasma cortisol when exercise in a hot environment is mild. Under the same conditions, the lack of heat acclimatization and dehydration can result in large plasma cortisol increases. When exercise is intense and core body temperature rises markedly, the plasma cortisol concentration increases during the initial days of heat acclimatization, but returns to control levels after 8 days of heat acclimatization, reflecting the reduction in total body strain. Physical training in a cool environment may or may not improve exercise economy. Metabolism can be affected by heat acclimatization, in that oxygen uptake during submaximal exercise is reduced.

Large effects have been reported for stair stepping; treadmill and cycle-ergometer exercise produce smaller, but statistically significant, changes. The physiologic mechanism has not been defined exactly, but three theories exist:

(a) blood flow to the skin increases, thus reducing central blood volume, venous return to the heart, and cardiac output;

(b) the portion of cardiac output perfusing muscle decreases; and

(c) the recruitment of muscle fibers shifts from predominantly oxidative to glycolytic fibers. Heat acclimatization reduces muscle glycogen utilization and post-exercise muscle lactate concentration.

Heat Illness

Heat acclimatization is of interest to physicians as well as athletes, because it reduces the incidence of heat illness and the intensity of symptoms. The most common heat illnesses among athletes are heat cramps, heat syncope, and heat exhaustion. Heat cramps are usually unheralded and occur in the voluntary muscles of the legs, arms, and abdomen, after several hours of strenuous exercise in individuals who have lost a large volume of sweat, have drunk a large volume of hypotonic fluid, and who have excreted a small volume of urine. Sodium depletion probably causes heat cramps. Heat acclimatization decreases the risk of experiencing heat cramps. Heat syncope (e.g., fainting) occurs most commonly during the first 3-5 days of heat exposure. This illness is related to the shunting of blood through dilated cutaneous vessels, postural pooling of blood, diminished venous return to the heart, reduction of cardiac output, and cerebral ischemia.

Heat syncope typically occurs when the ambient temperature or humidity rises suddenly, or when a non-acclimatized individual performs exercise in a hot environment. Heat acclimatization reduces the incidence of heat syncope to nearly zero, after 3-5 days of exercise-heat exposure. This period corresponds with cardiovascular stabilization, early in the course of heat acclimatization. Heat syncope is a syndrome distinct from heat exhaustion, because water and salt depletion do not always contribute to heat syncope. Heat exhaustion is the most commonly diagnosed form of heat illness among athletes, despite the fact that its symptoms are often vague and differ greatly from one situation to another.

Clinical descriptions include various combinations of headache, dizziness, fatigue, hyperirritability, tachycardia, hyperventilation, diarrhea, piloerection, hypotension, nausea, vomiting, syncope, heat cramps, as well as "heat sensations" in the head and upper torso. This explains why heat exhaustion is defined as the inability to continue exercise in a hot environment, and involves a diagnosis of exclusion. Heat acclimatization significantly reduces the signs and symptoms of heat exhaustion, after eight days of strenuous, intermittent running. The three aforementioned heat illnesses all involve either fluid-electrolyte balance, extracellular volume and tonicity, or cardiovascular adaptation. This emphasizes the importance of:

(a) ample dietary intake of NaCl and fluids, and

(b) fluid-electrolyte hormone regulation during heat acclimatization.

Factors affecting acclimatization

It is believed that host factors may influence the capacity to acclimatize to exercise in a hot environment. For example, older persons were previously thought to be less heat tolerant than their younger counterparts. Middle aged men (>45•yr) were shown to have higher heart rates, higher rectal temperatures, and lower sweat rates than young men, during exercise in the heat, both before and during exercise in the heat, both before and after heat acclimatization. Similarly, studies conducted in the late 1960s suggested that women were less tolerant of exercise in a hot environment than men. However, recent research has qualified and/or reversed these viewpoints. It is now recognized that few gender-related differences exist, when female and male subjects are matched for pertinent physical and morphological characteristics. It is also recognized that differences between older and younger subjects are not necessarily due to aging per se, but may be due to other factors such as decreased training volume and lower maximal aerobic power.

Most experts agree that intense physical training in a cool environment improves physiologic responses and speeds the process of heat acclimatization. During training in cool conditions, optimal physiologic adaptations may be achieved if strenuous interval training or continuous exercise, at an intensity above 50% of VO2max, is performed for 8-12 weeks. Maintenance of an elevated core body temperature appears to be the most important physiologic stimulus. Irrespective of physical training, VO2max generally influences physiologic responses during the development of heat acclimatization. Individuals with a high VO2max (>60 $ml.kg^{-1}.min^{-1}$) exhibit superior heart rate and rectal temperature responses, and usually reach a stable heat acclimatization state faster, when compared to those with a low VO2max (<40 $ml.kg^{-1}.min^{-1}$). However, maximal aerobic power per se may not be as important in conferring heat tolerance as the underlying physiologic adaptations (i.e. altered blood volume, vasodilation/ vasoconstriction, and muscle metabolism) which result in VO2max differences between individuals.

The phrase "heat intolerance" has been used in a wide variety of contexts. Interestingly, heat intolerance has been defined by some experts as an inability to develop normal physiologic adaptations, during repeated days of exercise in a hot environment. Some humans do not show the classic decreases in heart rate and rectal temperature that exemplify successful heat acclimatization. This has been of particular concern among persons with cardiovascular disease and prior heat stroke patients. One recent publication, however, reported that 9 out of 10 prior heat stroke patients exhibited normal heat acclimatization responses, 61 days after experiencing heatstroke.

Loss of acclimatization

The physiologic adaptations to exercise training in a cool environment are lost after several weeks or months of inactivity. In contrast, heat acclimatization adaptations may vanish after only a few days or weeks of inactivity (i.e., 18-28 days). The first adaptations to decay are those that develop first: heart rate and other cardiovascular variables. The rate of decay of adaptations is affected by the number of heat exposures per week, the number and format of training sessions, and the degree to which core body temperature is elevated. Athletes with high VO2max usually will lose heat acclimatization adaptations slower than individuals with low VO2max.

skin Infection

The skin plays an important role in protecting the body from noxious external stimuli such as mechanical forces, temperature changes, and harmful chemicals. It is no surprise, therefore, that cutaneous disorders are an important factor in every athletic specialty. Sports dermatology is concerned with skin disorders related to athletic activity, manifesting either as a primary disorder or as an exacerbation of a pre existing dermatological dermatosis. Sports dermatology is an enlarging field and this chapter summarizes some of the more commonly encountered problems.

Fungal infections

Dermatophytic fungi live in the stratum corneum (most superficial epidermal layer) and can cause superficial infections. Tinea pedis or 'athlete's foot' affects the interdigital and lateral areas of the feet and is characterized by pruritis, scaling, and occasional soreness. The classic 'wet form' presents with white macerated scale, fissures, and occasionally with vesicles and bullae. Less commonly a 'dry form' or 'moccasin foot' is seen as a dry, rough, diffuse white scale affecting the sole. The problem is often bilateral and the toenails may also be involved (manifest by discolouration, thickening, crumbling and Subungual scale of one or more toenails). Tinea pedis is a chronic disorder and patients may be afflicted for decades. Infection occurs by person-to-person or by contact with infected fomites such as a towel or floormat. It is undoubtedly influenced by the microenvironment of the clad foot, and factors which exacerbate the condition include a moist, warm environment; a sweaty foot enclosed in a non-absorbent sock and occlusive shoe such as a 'trainer' is a likely target for tinea pedis. Secondary bacterial infection is sometimes seen and may present as cellulitis, lymphangitis, or inguinal lymphadenopathy. The diagnosis of tinea pedis is confirmed by examining scrapings of keratinous debris in a 10% potassium hydroxide (KOH) preparation and observing the characteristic hyphae. Culture permits identification of the causative fungus.

The differential diagnosis includes pompholyx, pustular psoriasis, pitted keratolysis and allergic contact dermatitis to shoes; a positive skin scraping however does not necessarily exclude these dermatoses, as a superficial dermatophyte infection may be superimposed upon an area of already broken skin.

Treatment

Acutely inflamed 'wet' forms of superficial fungal infections should be treated with a combination of shooting antiseptic soaks or paints (e.g. Castellan's) and topical antifungals. Soaks should be lukewarm and contain potassium permanganate 1 in 10 000 and the feet immersed in the solution for 15 minutes three times daily. Effective topical antifungals include the newer imidaoles such as miconazole, econazole or clotrimoxazole in a cream or tincture base; these should be applied twice daily for approximately two weeks. Careful attention should be given to avoidance of exacerbating factors such as sweat, heat, and occlusion. Socks should be cotton or wool, and preferably changed once or twice during the day. Footwear such as thongs or clogs should be worn while using communal showers or change rooms.

Athletes should alternate pairs of sneakers or shoes if possible to allow airing in between periods of wear. Infection of the nails is an indication for oral antifungal therapy as dermatophyte in the nail are relatively resistant to topical agents. A new allylamine drug, terbinafine, can achieve a mycological cure of toenail onychomycosis in 70-80% of patients following twelve weeks of therapy. Other oral agents used include griseofulvin, ketoconazole and intermittent itraconazole. Although generally safe agents, ketoconazole is contraindicated in patients with hepatic disorders and can interact with other medications, for example, warfarin. Itraconazole has fewer hepatic side effects but is considerably more expensive than other oral antifungals. Amorolfine 5% nail lacquer can be applied to affected nails once or twice per week and has shown to cure approximately 40-55% of patients with toenail onychomycosis. Other fungal infections include tinea cruris, tinea versicolour and tinea incognita.

— *Tinea curis ('jock itch'):* Commences in the groin folds and extends out in an annular or circular fashion with a scaly, inflamed border. Hyphae can also be identified on KOH preparation of scale taken from the active advancing border. Treatment of tinea cruris is with oral griseofulvin and concomitant topical treatment with one of the newer imidazole creams.

— *Tinea versicolour:* Not actually a dermatophyte infection but is due to the saprophytic yeast Pityrosporum orbicular which develops into is parasitic fungal form Malasezia furfur. This transformation may be provoked by humidity, ambient heat, as a result of exercise, secondary to diabetes mellitus or iatrogenic immunosuppression e.g. systemic, corticosteroid treatment or immunosuppressives for solid organ transplants. Tinea versicolour infection produces hyper-or hypopigmented macules on the torso and proximal limbs with fine bran like scale. Infection can be chronic and recurrent with exacerbations following climatic changes in humidity. Organisms can be detected in a KOH preparation of skin scrapings.

Treatment of pityriasis versicolour has traditionally been with selenium sulphide applied as a cream to the affected areas twice daily or more recently with imidazole creams or foaming washes. Treatment needs to be applied to skin beyond the disappearance of the eruption, however, relapses are common with topical therapies. A course of oral ketoconazole or itraconazole for seven days is effective in eliminating the reservoir of Pityriasis organisms and helps prevent further relapses.

— *Tinea incognita:*Refers to the specific clinical picture seen when a potent topical corticosteroid preparation is mistakenly applied to a tinea infection. Inflammatory features such as erythema may be absent; typically a mild, pink, scaly annular macule with central clearing is seen. Skin scrapings stained with KOH show abundant hyphae and permit the correct diagnosis.

Bacterial infections

Impetigo

A superficial bacterial infection characterized by honey-coloured crusts or vesicles on a moist erythematous base. Impetigo is highly infectious and is spread by direct contact or fomites and can infect intact skin. The organism(s) responsible are usually streptococcus or staphylococcus aureus. High ambient temperatures, humidity, low altitude and poor hygiene may favour development and transmission of impetigo. Streptococcal impetigo has spread amongst footballers and those playing North American football.

Treatment consists of topical or systemic antibiotics directed against both streptococcus and staphylococcus. Removal of crusts by gentle soaking with warm compresses of potassium permanganate (1 in 10 000) dilution followed by a topical antibiotic such as mupirocin or fusidic acid, for approximately seven to ten days is effective. The entire skin, scalp included, should be washed with an antiseptic soap daily for ten days. Alternatively, a ten day course of broad spectrum oral antibiotics active against ß-lactamase producing staphylococci is also efficacious. The patient should be isolated until clearance of crusts and not allowed to compete in contact sports. In particular, sportsmen such as wrestlers should be free of new lesions for at least 48 hours prior to competition and should have no moist, exudative or draining lesions prior to tournament participation.

Pitted keratolysis

A bacterial infection of the palmar surface of the feet due to superficial infection with corynebacterium species. It characteristically appears as shallow white pits or dents in the stratum corneum. Increased sweating (hyperhidrosis) is thought to play an aetiological role in the condition and thus may be seen with increased frequency in athletes. Maceration and malodour may be associated findings.

Treatment consists of general preventative measures to control hyperhidrosis (absorbent socks, leather shoes, 'shoe-free' intervals), topical application of antiperspirants containing 20% aluminium chloride, an topical antibiotics such as 1-2% erythromycin or clindamycin solution.

Viral infections

Herpes simplex virus (HSV)

HSV is a double stranded DNA virus which typically causes recurrent infections of the mucous an periorifical membranes. However, it can infect any skin surface and remain latent in the ganglia of peripheral nerves.

Herpes gladiatorum

Herpes gladiatorum has been described in participants in

close contact sports such as wrestling and rugby (also known in the latter as 'scrumpox') and in a recent study of American college wrestlers 7.6% were reported to have had a herpes skin infection in the preceding 12 months1. Herpes gladiatorum is transmitted primarily by direct skin to skin contact, and abrasions in the skin may allow a pathway of infection.

The majority of lesions occur on the head or face, followed by the trunk and/or extremities. A prodromal itching or burning sensation is followed by clustered vesicular lesions on an erythematous base which heal with crusts over about one to three weeks. Less commonly headache, malaise, sore throat and fever may accompany the primary infection. Recurrent episodes may occur following the initial infection and may precipitated by sunburn, illness, and emotional stress.

HSV antibodies, acquired from previous cold sores, may be protective from acquiring herpes gladiatoraum eruptions. Because of its unexpected location on the cutaneous surface, herpes gladiatorum any be confused with impetigo, varicella, staphylococcal furunculosis, or allergic or irritant contact dermatitis. Adequate treatment, counseling and public health strategies depend on making an accurate diagnosis, hence viral immuno fluorescence and cultures should be obtained by gently breaking an intact vesicle and firmly rubbing the swab tip across the base of the erosion.

Treatment of herpes gladiatorum is ideally with oral acyclovir (200mg five times a day for the five days) and is most effective if commenced at the first symptoms of an outbreak. Topical acyclovir is available but is probably less effective. Concomitant secondary impetiginisation should also be treated. HSV can survive for hours to days outside the host if environmental conditions are appropriate2 hence all contaminated surfaces should be cleaned with antiseptic solution. In the vesicular phase and until the crusts have separated, patients should avoid sports which could involve physical contact.

Molluscum contagiosum

A highly infectious pox virus which can also be spread by human contact. The organism appears to be easily spread in an aqueous medium, for example, in communal baths, spas and pools. Amongst athletes, swimmers and cross country runners have the highest incidence of mollusca. Their incidence may be increased in patients with underlying active atopic dermatitis. They typically appear as solitary or multiple flesh-coloured dome shaped papules with a central umbilication. The differential diagnosis includes multiple basal cell carcinomata, cryptococcosis and appendageal tumours such as trichoepitheliomas. They can be treated by gently breaking the surface of the lesion and extracting the central keratinous plug. Other treatments employed are cryosurgery with liquid nitrogen, electrodessication and topical trichloroacetic acid or tretinoin. Athletes may resume contact sports 48 to 72 hours after the lesions have cleared.

Common warts

Are epidermal growths caused by infection by the human papillomavirus group (HPV). Infection can occur if infected debris from warts comes in contact with abraded skin and can result in either autoinoculation or transmission to susceptible individuals. However, it is not generally thought to be highly infective and thus not limit participation in contact sports. Plantar warts can cause pain with ambulation, thereby limiting performance in sporting activities. Warts may also be more common in callouses which develop in sport. Paring of plantar warts with a #15 blade reveals small black spots corresponding to thrombosed capillaries within papillae, thus distinguishing the lesions from callouses or corns, which lack these dots and have a central hyaline core.

Treatment of plantar warts is challenging and may cause as much inconvenience to the athlete as the presence of the wart itself. Daily application of salicylic and lactic acid preparations under occlusion with concomitant paring with an emery board may be effective, as may repeated cryosurgery and paring at two or three week intervals. For resistant warts, intralesional bleomycin injections or carbon dioxide ablation can be used. Oral high dose Cimetidine therapy (30-40mg/kg/day) has reportedly been successful in childhood warts; however other studies have shown no advantage in Cimetidine over placebo in adults.

Anabolic Steroids

Anabolic steroids (AS) are effective in enhancing athletic performance. The trade off, however, is the occurrence of adverse side effects which can jeopardize health. Since AS have effects on several organ systems, a myriad of side effects can be found. In general, the orally administered AS have more adverse effects than parenterally administered AS. In addition, the type of AS is not only important for the advantageous effects, but also for the adverse effects. Especially the AS containing a 17-alkyl group have potentially more adverse affects, in particular to the liver. One of the problems with athletes, in particular strength athletes and bodybuilders, is the use of oral and parenteral AS at the same time ("stacking"), and in dosages which may be several (up to 40 times) the recommended therapeutical dosage. The frequency and severity of side effects is quite variable. It depends on several factors such as type of drug, dosage, duration of use and the individual sensitivity and response.

Liver Function

AS may exert a profound adverse effect on the liver. This is particularly true for orally administered AS. The parenterally administered AS seem to have less serious effects on the liver. Testosterone cypionate, testosterone enanthate and other injectable anabolic steroids seem to have little adverse effects on the liver. However, lesions of the liver have been reported after parenteral nortestosterone administration, and also occasionally after injection of testosterone esters. The influence of AS on liver function has been studied extensively. The majority of the studies involve hospitalized patients who are treated for prolonged periods for various diseases, such as anemia, renal insufficiency, impotence, and dysfunction of the pituitary gland. In clinical trials, treatment with anabolic steroids resulted in a decreased hepatic excretory function. In addition, intra hepatic cholestasis, reflected by itch and jaundice, and hepatic peliosis were observed. Hepatic peliosis is a hemorrhagic cystic degeneration of the liver, which may lead to fibrosis and portal hypertension. Rupture of a cyst may lead to fatal bleeding.

. Benign (adenoma's) and malign tumors (hepatocellular carcinoma) have been reported. There are rather strong indications that tumors of the liver are caused when the anabolic steroids contain a 17-alpha-alkyl group.

Usually, the tumors are benign adenoma's, that reverse after stopping with steroid administration. However, there are some indications that administration of anabolic steroids in athletes may lead to hepatic carcinoma. Often these abnormalities remain asymptomatic, since peliosis hepatis and liver tumors do not always result in abnormalities in the blood variables that are generally used to measure liver function.

AS use is often associated with an increase in plasma activity of liver enzymes such as aspartate aminotransferase (AST), alanine aminotransferase (ALT), alkaline phosphatase (AP), lactate dehydrogenase (LDH), and gamma glutamyl transpeptidase (GGT). These enzymes are present in hepatocytes in relatively high concentrations, and an increase in plasma levels of these enzymes reflect hepatocellular damage or at least increased permeability of the hepatocellular membrane.

In longitudinal studies of athletes treated with anabolic steroids, contradictory results were obtained on the plasma activity of liver enzymes (AST, AST, LDH, GGT, AP). In some studies, enzymes were increased, whereas in others no changes were found. When increases were found, the values were moderately increased and normalized within weeks after abstinence. There are some suggestions that the occurrence of hepatic enzyme leakage, is partly determined by the pre-treatment condition of the liver. Therefore, individuals with abnormal liver function appear to be at risk.

Anabolic Steroids and the Male Reproductive System

AS are derivatives of testosterone, which has strong

genitotropic effects. For this reason, it will not be surprising that side effects include the reproductive system. Application of anabolic steroids leads to supra-physiological concentrations of testosterone or testosterone derivatives. Via the feed back loop, the production and release of luteinizing hormone (LH) and follicle stimulation hormone (FSH) is decreased. Prolonged use of anabolic steroids in relatively high doses will lead to hypogonadotrophic hypogonadism, with decreased serum concentrations of LH, FSH, and testosterone.

There are strong indications that the duration, dosage, and chemical structure of the anabolic steroids are important for the serum concentrations of gonadotropins. A moderate decrease of gonadotropin secretion causes atrophy of the testes, as well as a decrease of sperm cell production. Oligo, azoospermia and an increased number of abnormal sperm cells have been reported in athletes using AS, resulting in a decreased fertility. After stopping AS use, the gonadal functions will restore within some months. There are indications, however, that it may take several months. In bodybuilding, where usually high dosages are uses, after stopping steroid use, often choriogonadotropins are administered to stimulate testicular function. The effectiveness of this therapy is unknown.

The various studies suggest that using more than one type of anabolic steroid at the same time ("stacking") causes a stronger inhibition of the gonadal functions than using one single anabolic steroid. After abstention from anabolic steroids these changes in fertility usually reverse within some months. However, several cases of have been reported in which the situation of hypogonadism lasted for more than 12 weeks. A well known side effect of AS in males is breast formation (gynecomastia). Gynecomastia is caused by increased levels of circulating estrogens, which are typical female sex hormones. The estrogens estradiol and estrone are formed in males by peripheral aromatization and conversion of AS. The increased levels of circulation estrogens in males stimulate breast growth. In general, gynecomastia is irreversible.

AS may affect sexual desire. Although few investigations on this issue have been published, it appears that during AS use sexual desire is increased, although the frequency of erectile dysfunction is increased. This may seem contradictory, but sexual appetite is androgen dependent, while erectile function is not. Since sexual desire and aggressiveness are increased during AS use, the risk of getting involved in sexual assault may be increased.

Anabolic Steroids and the Female Reproductive System

In the normal female body small amounts of testosterone are produced, and as in males, artificially increasing levels by administration of AS will affect the hypothalamic-pituitary-gonadal axis. An increase in circulating androgens will inhibit the production and release of LH and FSH, resulting in a decline in serum levels of LH, FSH, estrogens and progesterone. This may result in inhibition of follicle formation, ovulation, and irregularities of the menstrual cycle. The irregularities of the menstrual cycle are characterized by a prolongation of the follicular phase, shortening of the luteal phase or amenorrhea. Although these changes are generally more pronounced in younger women, large inter-individual responsiveness to anabolic steroids exists. The effects of AS dosages as generally used in sport, on the hypothalamic-pituitary-gonadal axis in females are hardly studied.

Other side effects of anabolic steroid use in females are increased sexual desire and hypertrophy of the clitoris. The few systematic studies that have been conducted suggest that the effects are similar to the effects in patients, treated with anabolic steroids. Anabolic steroid use by pregnant women may lead to pseudohermaphroditism or to growth retardation of the female fetus. Anabolic steroid use may even lead to fetal death. However, these side effects have not been studied systematically. It is likely that the severity of the side effects is related to the dosage, duration of use and the type of the drug.

Additional side effects of anabolic steroids specifically in women are acne, hair loss, withdrawal of the frontal hair line, male pattern boldness, lowering of the voice, increased facial hair growth, and breast atrophy. The lowering of the voice, decreased breast size, clitoris hypertrophy and hair loss are generally irreversible. Females using AS may develop masculine facial traits, male muscularity, and coarsening of the skin. When anabolic steroids are administered in growing children side effects include virilization, gynecomastia, and premature closure of the epiphysis, resulting in cessation of longitudinal growth.

Cardiovascular System

AS also affect the cardiovascular system and the serum lipid profile. Relatively few studies have been done to investigate the effect of anabolic steroids on the cardiovascular system. No longitudinal studies have been conducted on the effect of anabolic steroids on cardiovascular morbidity and mortality. Most of the investigations have been focused on risk factors for cardiovascular diseases, and in particular the effect of anabolic steroids on blood pressure and on plasma lipoproteins. In most cross-sectional studies serum cholesterol and triglycerides between drug-free users and non-users is not different. However, during anabolic steroid use total cholesterol tends to increase, while HDL-cholesterol demonstrates a marked decline, well below the normal range.

Serum LDL-cholesterol shows a variable response: a slight increase or no change. The response of total cholesterol seems to be influenced by the type of training that is done by the athlete. When a great deal of the exercise consists of aerobic exercise, the increasing effect of AS is counterbalanced by an exercise-induced increasing effect, which may result in a net decline in total cholesterol. Aerobic training does not seem to be able to offset the steroid-induced decline in HDL-cholesterol and its subfractions HDL-2, and HDL-3. The precise effect of anabolic steroids on LDL-cholesterol is unknown yet. It appears that anabolic steroids influence hepatic triglyceride lipase (HTL) and lipoprotein lipase (LPL). Males usually have higher levels of HTL, while females have higher LPL activity. HTL is primarily responsible for the clearance of HDL-cholesterol, while LPL takes care of cellular uptake of free fatty acids and glycerol. Androgens and anabolic steroids stimulate HTL, presumably resulting in decreased serum levels of HDL-cholesterol. The effect of anabolic steroids on triglycerides is not well known. It is suggested that relatively low doses do not affect the serum triglyceride levels, while it cannot be excluded that higher doses elicit an increase.

No unanimity exists about the influence of anabolic steroids on arterial blood pressure. The response is most probably dose dependent. There is some data suggesting that high doses increase diastolic blood pressure, whereas low doses fail to have a significant effect on diastolic blood pressure. Increases in diastolic blood pressure normalize within 6-8 weeks after abstinence from anabolic steroids. It appears that repeated intermittent use of anabolic steroids does not affect diastolic blood pressure during drug free periods. There is evidence that the use of anabolic steroids does elicit structural changes in the heart and that the ischemic tolerance is decreased after steroid use.

Echocardiographic studies in bodybuilders, using anabolic steroids, reported a mild hypertrophy of the left ventricle, with a decreased diastolic relaxation, resulting in a decreased diastolic filling. Some investigators have associated cardiomyopathy, myocardial infarction, and cerebro-vascular accidents with abuse of anabolic steroids. However, a possible causal relationship could not been proved, because longitudinal studies that are necessary to prove such a relationship, have not been conducted yet. There is convincing evidence that oral administration of anabolic steroids has stronger adverse effects on the mentioned variables than parenteral administration.

Although the effects of anabolic steroids have an unfavorable influence on the risk factors for cardiovascular disease, no data are available about the long term effects. Most of the mentioned effects appear to reverse within 6-8 weeks after abstention. It is unknown, however, whether the structural changes as reported in the heart, are reversible as well.

Psychological Effects

Administration of AS may affect behavior. Increased testosterone levels in the blood are associated with masculine behavior, aggressiveness and increased sexual desire. Increased aggressiveness may be beneficial for athletic training, but may also lead to overt violence outside the gym or the track. There are reports of violent, criminal behavior in individuals taking AS. Other side effects of AS are euphoria, confusion, sleeping disorders, pathological anxiety, paranoia, and hallucinations. Anabolic steroid users may become dependent on the drug, with symptoms of withdrawal after cessation of drug use.

The withdrawal symptoms consist of aggressive and violent behavior, mental depression with suicidal behavior, mood changes, and in some cases acute psychosis. At present it is unknown which individuals are particularly at risk. It is likely that great individual differences in responsiveness may exist. Some individuals try to minimize the withdrawal affects by administration of human choriogonadotropins (hCG), in order to enhance endogenous testosterone production. However, it is unknown in how far the hCG administration is successful in ameliorating the withdrawal effects.

Additional Side Effects

In addition to the mentioned side effects several others have been reported. In both males and females acne are frequently reported, as well as hypertrophy of sebaceous glands, increased tallow excretion, hair loss, and alopecia. There is some evidence that anabolic steroid abuse may affect the immune system, leading to a decreased effectiveness of the defense system. Steroid use decreases the glucose tolerance, while there is an increase in insulin resistance. These changes mimic Type II diabetes. These changes seem to be reversible after abstention from the drugs. There are some case reports suggesting a causal relationship between anabolic steroid use and the occurrence of Wilms tumor, and prostatic carcinoma. In the literature also sleep apnea has been reported, which has been associated with AS-induced increased in hematocrit, leading to blood stasis and thrombosis.

AS use may affect thyroid function. Administration of AS has been found to decrease thyroid stimulation hormone (TSH), and the products of the thyroid gland. In addition, thyroid binding globulin (TBG). These changes reversed within weeks after discontinuation of AS use. A serious consequence of AS use may be the multiple drug abuse. On the one hand athletes use different kinds of drugs in an attempt to counterbalance the side effects: hCG, thyroid hormones, anti-estrogens, anti-depressants. On the other hand people try to support the anabolic effects of AS by using additional anabolic hormones as for instance: different types of AS at the same time, growth hormone, insulin, erythropoietine, and clenbuterol. Because most of this takes place outside the official medical circuit, it is likely that these practices may lead to serious conditions.

5

Exercise and Sports Nutrition

Exercise training is an adaptive process. The body will adapt to the stress of exercise with increased fitness if the stress is above a minimum threshold intensity. To achieve maximum effectiveness, we must consider factors involved in the adaptation of muscle to stress and deconditioning. These factors include overload, specificity, reversibility, and individual differences. An interesting aspect of skeletal muscle is its adaptability. If a muscle is stressed (within tolerable limits), it adapts and improves its function. For example, weight lifters exercise their arms and shoulders, so their muscles hypertrophy and improve their strength. Larger muscles allow them to accommodate an increased load. Likewise, if a muscle receives less stress than it's used to, it atrophies. For example, the muscles of a casted leg atrophy in response to disuse.

The purpose of physical training is to stress systematically the body so it improves its capacity to exercise. Physical training is beneficial only as long as it forces the body to adapt to the stress of physical effort. If the stress is not sufficient to overload the body, then no adaptation occurs. If a stress cannot be tolerated, then injury or over-training results. Significant improvements in performance occur when the appropriate exercise stresses are introduced into the athlete's training program. Physical fitness is largely a reflection of the level of training. When an athlete is working hard, fitness is high. However, when heavy training ceases, fitness begins to deteriorate. There are countless exercise devices and training programs available that are hailed as the best way to gain strength. In most instances, as long as a threshold tension is developed, increases in strength will occur.

The type of strength developed is the important consideration in exercise and sports. Long distance running up steep hills, for example, will develop a certain amount of muscular strength. The muscular adaptations that result will differ from those produced from high resistance, low repetition squats (knee bends). The distance runner develops mainly sarcoplasmic protein (oxidative enzymes, mitochondrial mass, etc.), while the weight lifter develops mainly contractile protein. The nature of the adaptive response must always be considered when designing the training program. Factors that determine the rate and type of strength gains include overload, specificity, and reversibility.

Muscles increase their strength and size when they are forced to contract at tensions close to their maximum. Muscles must be overloaded to hypertrophy and improve strength. Experimental and empirical observations have allowed generalizations concerning the amount of overload necessary for strength gains. Muscle protein accumulation occurs by increasing the rate of protein synthesis, decreasing the rate of protein degradation, or both. Fiber types differ in their response to overload. Slow fibers hypertrophy by decreasing the rate of protein degradation. Fast fibers hypertrophy by increasing the rate of protein synthesis. The rate of protein synthesis in a muscle is directly related to the rate of entry of amino acids into the cells. Amino acid transport into muscle is influenced directly by the intensity and duration of muscle tension. This was determined by experiments with isolated muscle. They were bathed in a solution containing labeled amino acids, such as 14C labeled a-amino isobutyric acid. It was found that amino acid uptake was highest when muscles were contracted. Uptake was greater as tension and the duration of tension increased. Weight training studies and empirical observations of athletes have reinforced the importance of generating muscular tension. It must be developed at an adequate intensity and duration for the optimal development of strength.

The majority of studies have found that the ideal number of repetitions are between four and eight (repetitions maximum, 4-8 RM). They should be practiced in multiple sets (3 or more). Strength gains are less when either fewer or greater numbers of repetitions are used. These findings are consistent with the progressive resistance training practices of athletes. Athletes involved in speed-strength sports practice low repetition, high intensity exercise during or immediately preceding the competitive season. These athletes include shot-putters and discus throwers. Such training improves explosive strength, while allowing sufficient energy reserves for practicing motor skills. However, the effectiveness of this practice has not been established experimentally.

Body builders usually do more sets and repetitions of exercises and more exercises per body part than weight lifters or strength athletes. Their goal is to build large, defined, symmetrical muscles. It is not known if typical body building training method is the most effective means of achieving their goals. Numerous studies have shown that high resistance, low repetition exercises are more effective than low resistance, high repetition exercises in promoting muscle hypertrophy. Proper rest intervals are important for maximizing tension, both between exercises and training sessions. Insufficient rest results in inadequate recovery and a diminished capacity of the muscle to exert full force. Unfortunately, the ideal rest interval between exercises has not been determined. Most athletes strength train three to four days per week with large muscle exercises, such as the squat and bench press, rarely done more than twice a week. This practice has been empirically derived. It allows adequate recovery between training sessions.

The overload must be progressively increased for consistent gains in strength to occur. However, because of the high dangers of over-training in strength building exercises, constantly increasing the resistance is sometimes counter-productive. A relatively new practice among strength trained athletes is periodization of training. This practice varies the volume and intensity of exercises so the nature of the exercise stress frequently changes. Many athletes believe that this practice produces a faster rate of adaptation. Periodization of training will be discussed further in the section on the progressive resistance training programs of athletes.

Specificity

Muscles adapt specifically to the nature of the exercise stress. The progressive resistance training program should stress the muscles how they are to perform. The most obvious example of specificity is that the muscle exercised is the muscle that adapts to training. Thus, if you exercise the leg muscles, they hypertrophy rather than the muscles of the shoulders. There is specific recruitment of motor units within a muscle depending upon the requirements of the contraction . The different muscle fiber types have characteristic contractile properties. The slow twitch fibers are relatively fatigue-resistant, but have a lower tension capacity than the fast twitch fibers. The fast twitch fibers can contract more rapidly and forcefully, but they also fatigue rapidly. The use of a motor unit is dependent on the threshold levels of its alpha motor neuron. The low threshold, slow twitch fibers are recruited for low intensity activities such as jogging (and for that matter, most tasks of human motion). However, for high speed or high intensity activities, such as weight lifting, the fast twitch motor units are recruited.

The amount of training that occurs in a muscle fiber is determined by the extent that it is recruited. High repetition, low intensity exercise, such as distance running, uses mainly slow twitch fibers. Endurance training improves the fibers' oxidative capacity. Low repetition, high intensity activity, such as weight training, causes hypertrophy of fast twitch fibers. There are some changes to the lower threshold slow twitch fibers. The training program should be structured to produce the desired training effect. Increases in strength are very specific to the type of exercise, even when the same muscle groups are used.

Specific motor units are recruited for specific tasks. If a person is weight training to improve strength for another activity, the exercises should be as close as possible to desired movements. Likewise, when attempting to increase strength after an injury or surgery, rehabilitation should include muscle movements as close as possible to normal activities.

Muscle fiber type appears to play an important role in determining success in some sports. Successful distance runners have a high proportion of slow twitch muscles (percent slow twitch fibers is highly related to maximum oxygen consumption). Sprinters have a predominance of fast twitch muscles. Several studies have shown that a high content of fast twitch fibers is a prerequisite for success in progressive resistance training. This is understandable, as the fast twitch fibers experience selective hypertrophy as a result of high resistance, low repetition exercise. However, all sports do not require prerequisite fiber characteristics. For example, in world class shot-putters there is a surprisingly diverse muscle fiber composition. In those athletes, larger muscle fibers rather than percent fiber type, accounted for their performance.

There are differences in the relative percentage of fast twitch fibers in explosive strength athletes. Having a high percentage of fast-twitch fibers is not necessary critical for success. Many strength athletes have a higher fast-to-slow twitch fiber area ratio than in sedentary subjects and endurance athletes. Individual differences in training intensity and technique can make up for deficiencies in the relative percentage of fast twitch fibers in these athletes. It would be interesting to speculate about the performance of a shot-putter with a high percentage of fast twitch fibers. What would performance be like in an athlete who developed good strength and technique? The high percentage of fast twitch fibers would probably be a decided advantage.

Simultaneous participation in a training program designed to stimulate both strength and endurance has been found to interfere with gains in strength. Strength athletes may inhibit their ability to gain strength by participating in vigorous endurance activities. Muscles may be unable to adapt optimally to both forms of exercise.

Reversibility

Muscles will atrophy as a result of disuse, immobilization, and starvation. Muscles adapt to increasing levels of stress by increasing their function. Disuse leads to decreasing strength and muscle mass. Atrophy results in a decrease in both contractile and sarcoplasmic protein. The muscle fiber types do not atrophy at the same rate. Joint immobilization results in a faster rate of atrophy for the slow twitch muscle. This has important implications for rehabilitation. Often, increasing strength is a major goal following immobilization. Endurance should also be stressed because of the relatively greater loss of slow twitch muscle capacity.

Immobilization affects muscle length. If a muscle is fixed in a lengthened position, sarcomeres are added, while they are lost if the muscle is immobilized in a shortened position. Immobilization also leads to a variety of biochemical changes including decreased glycogen, adenosine diphosphate (ADP), creatine phosphate (CP),and creatine. All of these factors can affect muscular performance after immobilization has ended.

As with other forms of exercise, people vary in the rate they gain strength. Some of these differences can be attributed to the relative predominance of fast- and slow-twitch motor units in muscles. Usually, endurance athletes will have a more slow twitch fibers in their active muscles. Strength athletes will have more fast twitch fibers. Intense progressive resistance training mainly enlarges fast-twitch fibers. People who have more fast-twitch fibers will tend to gain strength faster than those who do not. Muscle strength is related to the cross-sectional area of the muscle. However, this strong relationship diminishes when "explosive athletes" and endurance athletes are compared. What most studies suggest is that strength is highly related to muscle size. However, people who have a disproportionate amount of fast-twitch fibers will gain strength faster than those who do not. Fast-twitch fibers tend to be stronger than other fiber types, so people who have more of them will tend to be stronger and have greater potential for strength gains. Several studies have shown that fiber composition is genetically determined. Genetic researchers often investigate the influence of heritability on a trait by studying monozygotic and dizygotic twins (identical and nonidentical twins). Fiber distribution and muscle enzyme activity in monozygotic twins is almost identical in most of these studies.

Genetics is not the sole determinant of individual differences in strength. Numerous studies have shown that many successful strength-speed athletes do not have a predominance of fast-twitch motor units in critical muscles. Further, in athletic subjects, fiber composition is only marginally related to the time subjects can maintain isometric force and perform explosive squat jumps. Genetics exert a strong influence on the ability to gain strength. A good training program can make up for "genetic deficiencies."

Adaptation is the whole purpose of exercise training. Adaptation requires a systematic application of exercise stress. The stress should be sufficient to stimulate an adaptation, but not so severe that breakdown and injury occur.

Why is sports nutrition important and who is it important for? It is easy to understand the search for a competitive edge in the elite world of sport. In many events, the margin between winning and losing is measured in millimetres and hundredths of seconds, and the stakes include international fame and considerable amounts of money. A number of prominent sports scientists have suggested that at this level, where genetics, training, equipment and motivation are all equalized, nutrition might provide the vital ingredient in success. However, it is clear that recreational athletes are also interested in sports nutrition, as shown by the recent boom in the marked for specialized sports drinks and sports bars. Although some people consider that special sports nutrition strategies are relevant only to the elite athlete (or that these specialized sports foods are a waste of money for the non-elite sportsperson), it is important to realize that the fundamentals of exercise physiology apply to sporting activities, regardless of the talent of the athlete involved. For example, sweat losses and carbohydrate needs are created by muscular activity. While for recreational athletes, the rewards of sports nutrition strategies are likely to be the satisfaction of improving 'personal bests' or achieving personal goals, the spin-off of better safety and enjoyment of exercise activities may be an important factor in encouraging population participation in exercise.

Finally, since many of the principles of sports nutrition concur with population dietary guidelines, the interest in sports nutrition may independently help to improve the general health and nutritional status of the population. Sports nutrition is underpinned by the sciences of exercise physiology and biochemistry, and aims to supply the body with the nutrients needed to adapt to a training program, to perform optimally during competition and to recover quickly after exercise. However, sports nutrition also involves the art of translating nutrient needs into foods and eating practices that are compatible with the busy schedule and commitments of an athlete's lifestyle.

The purpose of training is to prepare the athlete to perform at their best during key competitions, and inmost situations the time and demands of this preparation far outweigh those of competition. Therefore, it is the everyday or training diet of the athlete which has the greatest impact on sports performance. The athlete shares the population nutritional goals of meeting nutrient requirements for immediate health, as well as adopting dietary strategies to reduce the risk of developing Western disease patterns in later life. Additionally, they should be able to participate in the enjoyment and social interaction that is provided by food. However, the athlete must also meet special goals of sports nutrition during the training phase including:

— to achieve a body size and composition that is ideal for performance in the athlete's sport

— to meet additional demands for energy and nutrients that arise from the training program

— to undertake dietary strategies that optimize performance during training sessions and enhance recovery after the session

— to practice any competition nutrition strategies in advance so that these can be fine-tuned for success.

The importance and the details of these goals will vary from sport to sport.

The size, shape and composition of the body are important determinants of performance in many sports. In some sports, weight divisions or limits are set to encourage fair competition between opponents of equal size and strength. These sports include weight lifting, boxing, judo, light weight rowing and horse racing. In other sports, a low weight and/or low body weight level is a factor in successful performance. This may be to increase the athlete's 'power to weight' ratio, or to reduce 'dead weight' that must be transported over long distances (e.g. in distance running, road cycling or triathlons) or moved against gravity (e.g. jumping events, hill cycling). In some sports, the aesthetic appeal of a lean body provides favourable characteristics for judging (e.g. in body building, gymnastics, figure skating), although this is usually combined with the biomechanical advantages of being small and light (e.g. in gymnastics).

In many situations, the athlete achieves a suitable body size and shape for their sport as a result of the combination of the genetics which have 'selected' them to excel in that sport in the first place, and their training programme. However in other situations the athlete may desire to alter their physique - typically to lose body fat or to gain muscle mass.

Reducing weight and body fat

Sometimes the need to lose body fat is desirable and achievable. Some athletes become overfat due to poor dietary intake (e.g. as a result of poor nutrition knowledge or erratic eating patterns due to travel) or due to a period of a low energy expenditure (e.g. during the off-season, or while injured). These athletes can be assisted by changes to nutrition, training and lifestyle to regain their 'optimal' body fat level. In general, body fat losses are achieved by a sustained program of moderate energy restriction and appropriate training/increased energy expenditure. However there is much concern about athletes who seek to achieve body weight and fat goals that are extreme and unnatural. There is considerable pressure on athletes in many sports to achieve very low body fat levels in the belief that 'less is better', or to achieve body fat and weight standards that are arbitrarily set by coaches or other authorities.

These practices do not allow for individual variability in physique, nor do they encourage safe and healthy methods to achieve loss of weight and body fat. This situation is particularly true for female endurance athletes, whose desired body fat levels often seem below the 'natural' level for the individual, despite their heavy training programme. The problem is compounded in the case of females in 'aesthetic' sports (e.g. gymnasts and figure skaters), where training is skill-based and energy balance must be changed primarily through energy restriction. Problems also occur in weight division sports where the tradition is to compete in a weight class which is considerably below 'normal' training weight, and to 'make weight' by 'dieting' to reduce body fat levels, superimposed by acute dehydration during the day(s) prior to the event. Performance in 'weight making' sports is likely to be impaired due to the effects of fuel depletion and dehydration. However, in the larger view there appears to be an increased risk of disordered eating and eating disorders among athletes in sports in which low body fat levels are emphasized. It is a challenge of sports nutrition to assist athletes to set and achieve body weight and body fat goals that are truly 'ideal'. This should include the notion of individuality, allowing the goals to be set according to the athlete's history and realistic potential. Studies of elite sports show that, although there is a 'typical' physique that seems favourable for performance, there is considerable variation in the physique of well-performing athletes.

The athlete should be aware of the disadvantages of fad diets and of extreme fat/weight loss techniques. They should also recognize that there may be penalties for achieving very low body fat levels, at least when it does not seem to be penalties for achieving very low body fat levels, at least when it does not seem to be the athlete's natural physique. These include hormonal, physiological and psychological disturbances and may result from the low body fat level itself, as well as from the methods involved in achieving it (i.e. restricted eating, overtraining, stress). An 'ideal' weight and body fat level for any athlete should guarantee consistently good performances over a long term period, promote good health, and allow the athlete to consume a diet of sufficient energy and nutrients that allows all goals of training to be achieved. The need for individualized and expert advice on management of body weight and fat is the most common reason for an athlete to seek the services of a sports dietitian.

Increasing muscle mass

The other physique change desired by athletes is an increase in muscle size and strength. This is principally achieved by a suitable resistance training programme and genetic potential; however an adequate energy intake and usually, a positive energy balance is required. Although the protein needs for optimal muscle gain remain an emotive area for many athletes (and scientists), the primary dietary requirement for gain in muscle mass is energy. For some athletes, dietary counseling is required to provide strategies for increasing energy intake in an already high energy diet or in a busy timetable.

The energy requirements of athletes vary markedly and are influenced by the size of the athlete, the need to lose or gain weight, growth, and the training load (frequency, duration and intensity). However, while the energy requirements of female athletes might reasonably be - 20-30% lower than their male counterparts, principally to take smaller size into account, some surveys of female athletes often report an 'energy imbalance' whereby reported intakes of 4-8 MJ/day (1000-2000 Cal/day) are lower than expected and sometimes do not seem to cover the costs of the training programme itself. There appears to be no physiological explanation for this. Rather, systematic under reporting of food intake or 'restricted' eating during the period of the food diary due to concerns about body fat levels are suspected.

Protein needs of athletes

The protein requirements of athletes are increased by training. This results from the small contribution of protein oxidation to the fuel requirements of exercise as well as the protein needed to support muscle gain and repair of damaged body tissues. While athletes undertaking recreational or light training activities will meet their protein needs within population protein RDIs, a guideline for increased protein intake for heavily training athletes, both endurance and strength-training, has been set at 1.2-

1.6 g/kg BM/day. These targets are easily met within the increased energy requirement enjoyed by athletes who undertake such training. Indeed most dietary surveys show that athletes who eat a typical mixed diet report protein intakes within or above these goals. Despite this evidence, many body builders and weightlifters eat unnecessarily large amounts of protein-rich foods or buy expensive protein supplements.

6

Anterior Cruciate Ligament Prostheses

There are several approaches to treating severe knee ligament injuries, including non-operative management, primary repair, and surgical reconstruction using biological grafts or synthetic prostheses. Collateral ligament injuries heal well with conservative treatment or surgical repair. In contrast, surgical reconstruction is recommended for cruciate ligament tears, due to their poor intrinsic healing potential. The anterior cruciate ligament (ACL) is injured more frequently and has been studied much more extensively than the posterior cruciate ligament (PCL). Although significant progress has been made toward understanding the anatomy, composition, biomechanics, and healing of the ACL, there is still no graft or prosthesis ideally suited for ACL reconstruction.

Initial Mechanical Properties of ACL Prostheses

The ACL is considered to be the primary mechanical link between the femur and the tibia, so its mechanical properties-are crucial to its function. The mechanical behavior of the ACL is complex, with variable tension among fiber bundles, variable modulus as a function of load level, viscoelastic effects (creep, relaxation, strain-rate sensitivity), etc., which are discussed elsewhere. Here, the ultimate mechanical properties (e.g., breaking load and stiffness; tensile strength and modulus) of the ACL and prostheses are considered.

The ACL has considerable strength and modulus due to an aligned type I collagen network that bears great loads while undergoing little deformation. Breaking loads of 1725-2160 N have been reported for young human ACLs. The tensile strength of the human ACL is at least 38 MPa. The ultimate mechanical properties of ligaments generally increase during development, then decrease with aging. Various synthetic materials have been used either as 'permanent' ACL prostheses, tissue ingrowth devices, or graft augmentation devices.

The first generation of ACL prostheses had very poor initial mechanical properties. Today, prostheses can be fabricated with more appropriate initial mechanical properties, equaling or exceeding the properties of the normal human ACL. For example, the Gore-Tex ligament has a breaking load of 4800 N. Regardless of their initial mechanical properties, however, most permanent ligament prostheses still perform poorly in the long-term. Furthermore, the initial mechanical properties of the reconstructed bone-ligament-bone (BLB) complex depend on other factors besides the mechanical properties of the prosthesis - the method of surgical fixation to the bones is a limiting factor.

Effect of surgical fixation

Although the mechanical properties of the prosthesis are important, the initial mechanical properties of the reconstructed BLB complex are limited by the method of surgical fixation to the femur and tibia. The freshly reconstructed BLB complex consistently fails at the osseous attachment sites, not in the midsubstance of the prosthesis. Typically, surgical bone tunnels are made for fixation at the anatomic ACL attachment sites, although some have argued that over-the-top fixation can be biomechanically equivalent or superior to anatomic tunnel fixation.

Prostheses can be attached to bone using sutures, staples, screws, washers, and combinations of these methods. Simple suture or staple fixation fails at very low loads, less than 200 N. Screws with washers or plates perform better, failing at loads of about 200-250 N. A double 'locking ligament' suture fails near 400 N; when reinforced with a staple the failure load exceeds 400 N. Some ACL prostheses have plugs on the ends, resembling bone plugs, and are fixed within the bone tunnel using interference screws, similar to patellar tendon grafts. The strength of this type of fixation is heavily dependent on the quality of bone and bone compression.

In short, surgical fixation is a weak link that severely limits the initial mechanical properties of the reconstructed BLB complex. Thus, even if a prosthesis has a breaking load exceeding 2000 N, the initial breaking load of the reconstructed BLB complex may be only 25% of that value, about 450 N.

Several other surgical factors strongly influence the initial and long-term results of ACL reconstruction. For example, bone tunnel placement and initial tension on the implant must be carefully controlled to achieve consistent results. Determination of the best values for these and other surgical variables, to optimize knee biomechanics following ACL reconstruction, continues to be an important and active field of orthopedic research.

Post-Surgical Changes in Prosthetic Ligaments

Synthetic polymers evaluated clinically for ACL reconstruction include polytetrafluoroethylene (Gore-Tex), polyethylene terephthalate (Dacron; Stryker-Meadox and Leeds-Keio ligaments), carbon fibers (Integraft), and braided polypropylene (Kennedy Ligament Augmentation Device). Although several synthetic ACL prostheses are conditionally approved by the United States Food and Drug Administration (FDA) for salvage cases, or as graft augmentation devices, no prosthesis is unconditionally approved for primary ACL reconstruction. Experimental and clinical ACL reconstruction studies have generally shown poor long-term results due to persistent pain, synovitis, sterile effusions, arthritis, and mechanical breakdown of the synthetic polymers.

Permanent Prostheses

A permanent synthetic prosthesis that does not receive host tissue ingrowth is prone to long-term mechanical failure in the joint. Potential mechanical problems associated with permanent synthetic prostheses include creep (gradual stretching under load) and fatigue failure due to cyclic loading. Furthermore, the prosthesis may fray or rupture at the sharp bone tunnel attachment sites. Then, prosthesis fragments or wear debris particles may accelerate damage to the surrounding tissues. The Gore-Tex prosthetic ligament is composed of braided bundles of polytetrafluoroethylene (PTFE), an inert polyethylene with fluorine substituted for hydrogen side groups. The failure load of the prosthesis is 4830 N and the stiffness is 322 N/mm. The Gore-Tex device performed well as a permanent ACL prosthesis in 15 month clinical trials, improving knee stability in 129 out of 130 patients. In 1986, the FDA conditionally approved the Gore-Tex ligament prosthesis to salvage failed autografts, sparing the patient from a total knee replacement procedure. Clinical trials using the device for ACL reconstruction continue to be reported, and the results seem to deteriorate with time. In two-year clinical trials, 87% of the patients had satisfactory results, but 4 of 39 prostheses had ruptured. In a 3 year study, the Gore-Tex prosthesis performed poorly due to sterile effusions and persistent pain in 6 out of 18 patients. The probability of survival of the prosthesis decreased sharply from 2 to 5 years post-implantation, and the overall failure rate of the Gore-Tex prosthesis was 33%. In 268 patients with average follow-up of 4 years, unacceptable results were reported in 56% of the patients; effusions occurred in 34% of the patients, and the device ruptured in 12% of the patients.

Permanent ACL prostheses have also been made from Dacron (polyethylene terephthalate), a polyester with a rigid aromatic ring incorporated into the backbone chain. The Stryker-Meadox Dacron ACL prosthesis was not approved by the FDA for ACL reconstruction. Using a modified Macintosh procedure and augmentation of the Dacron prosthesis with iliotibial band, a 60% failure rate was found at a mean follow-up time of almost 4 years. Five of 40 Dacron prostheses (12.5%) had ruptured by this time. At 5 years follow-up, 23% of unaugmented Dacron prostheses had ruptured. Similarly, 28% of Dacron prostheses had ruptured at an average follow up of 4.4 years in another study. This study was particularly disturbing because degenerative arthritis was found in the patients with the ruptured prostheses, perhaps due to wear debris. Others reported overall failure rates of 20% at 2 years increasing to 35.7% at 5 years follow-up for permanent Dacron ACL prostheses.

The results of ACL reconstruction deteriorate with time for both Gore-Tex and Dacron permanent prostheses. Permanent ACL prostheses that do not induce supportive tissue ingrowth will likely fail in the long-term, due to synovitis, effusions, arthritis, or mechanical deterioration of the prosthesis.

Non-Degradable Scaffolds Designed for Tissue In growth

Tissue ingrowth or scaffolding devices for ACL reconstruction have been developed from several types of polymers, including Dacron and carbon fibers. These devices are designed with a porous or filamentous structure to promote host neoligament tissue ingrowth. The amount of host tissue ingrowth depends more on the mechanical properties and surface morphology than the chemical composition of the implant. The implanted scaffold should provide mechanical support and promote ingrowth of host neoligament tissue. Mechanical loads should be transferred gradually from the implanted scaffold to the neoligament tissue.

The Leeds-Keio synthetic ligament, composed of a Dacron mesh, was designed as a scaffolding structure to support host tissue ingrowth. The inventors of this device have reported successful clinical results, with arthroscopic observations documenting neoligament tissue development within the implanted Dacron scaffold. Other investigators, however, reported nonaligned fibrous tissue, not true neoligament tissue, ingrown within the device after implantation in a sheep model. They suggested that the Leeds-Keio ligament did not serve as a true scaffolding device, but instead behaved as a permanent load-bearing prosthesis, subject to long-term failure in the joint.

Filamentous carbon has also been used to develop a scaffolding device to induce neotendon and neoligament tissue ingrowth. Implants consist of approximately 10,000 individual fibers, each with a diameter of about 10 mm. The individual fibers have very high tensile strength (2100-2350 MPa), but are brittle, resulting in fiber fracture and the release of potentially harmful debris. A resorbable polymeric coating was somewhat successful in preventing carbon fiber breakage and localizing debris. However, due to poor performance and permanent wear debris in the joint, the Integraft carbon fiber device was not approved by the FDA for ACL reconstruction. In theory, a tissue ingrown device, unlike a permanent prosthesis, should remodel in response to long-term mechanical loads. Although the concept is interesting, there have been problems in implementing this design.

Tissue ingrowth may be delayed, or may occur only in limited amounts. Even if ingrowth is substantial, the tissue can be disorganized and weak, resembling scar tissue instead of neoligament tissue. If the stiffness of the implant greatly exceeds that of the ingrown host tissue, most of the mechanical load will be borne by the implant, and the load-deprived host tissue will not remodel or mature. This phenomenon of stress-shielding is a major concern for both tissue ingrowth devices and graft augmentation devices.

Graft-Augmentation Devices

Graft augmentation devices were developed to protect biological grafts from high loads in the early postoperative period of graft weakness. These devices are normally implanted in parallel with a biological graft (autograft or allograft) to share the mechanical loads. The amount of load borne by each component is proportional to its stiffness. Therefore, the device stiffness should approximate that of the biological graft to avoid stress-shielding.

Dacron has been used as a graft augmentation device in addition to being used as a permanent prosthesis and a tissue ingrowth device. The Dacron device reportedly shielded autogenous grafts from bearing mechanical loads, resulting in poor long-term neoligament development in augmented grafts compared to unaugmented grafts. Stress-shielding continues to be a major concern for graft augmentation devices, and tissue ingrowth devices as well. To address the problem of stress-shielding by stiff synthetic polymers, investigators augmented patellar tendon autografts in primates using the Gore-Tex ACL prosthesis placed in an over-the-top position (nonparallel, nonisometric).

The device was implanted this way to provide increased protection to the graft as the knee was extended. Knee laxity was decreased by this augmentation procedure, and autograft incorporation and remodeling occurred at similar rates for augmented and control groups. The Kennedy LAD (ligament augmentation device) is a braided polypropylene yarn with an initial breaking load of about 1500 N and a stiffness of 36 N/mm. The stiffness of the Kennedy LAD is low, and the device is attached to bone on only one end of the autogenous repair. Due to the low stiffness of the device, stress-shielding of the graft is reduced, so normal neoligament remodeling should occur. Patellar tendon allografts in sheep had improved initial strength and stability in LAD-augmented knees. In the long-term, the biomechanical properties of augmented and unaugmented allografts were similar, suggesting that normal tissue remodeling occurred in the presence of the augmentation device. Clinical results using this LAD were promising, and the FDA conditionally approved the device only for augmentation of a Marshall Macintosh ACL reconstruction procedure. However, investigators recently reported no difference in the clinical outcome for augmented and unaugmented semitendinosus tendon autografts at about 2 years follow-up. An augmentation device is needed only temporarily, to share mechanical loads with the biological graft, so long-term maintenance of the mechanical properties of the device is not necessary or even desirable. Ideally, graft augmentation devices should be resorbable, gradually transferring mechanical loads completely to the biological graft.

Fibroblast-Seeded Scaffolds

In vitro 'seeding' of viable fibroblasts within the scaffold implant may stimulate early healing and improve neoligament formation. Fibroblasts play a major role in collagen turnover during healing and tissue remodeling. Furthermore, fibroblast function depends on the source or type of fibroblast. For example, fibroblasts from the ACL and medial collateral ligament have different intrinsic capacities for migration and proliferation. Ligament analogs consisting of collagen scaffolds seeded with extra- or intra- articular fibroblasts have different healing potentials in vitro depending on the fibroblast source. These fibroblast-seeded collagen scaffolds should be a useful tool to explore the role of different fibroblast types in neoligament formation. The clinical goal is to promote early healing and improve long-term remodeling and biomechanical performance in the reconstructed ACL by using ligament analogs (fibroblast-seeded scaffolds) instead of biological grafts or synthetic prostheses.

The long-term biomechanical performance of ACL prostheses is unsatisfactory. Permanent ACL prostheses are prone to creep, fatigue, and mechanical failure within several years after implantation. Tissue ingrowth scaffolds and ligament augmentation devices require further refinement to provide effective mechanical support while avoiding stress-shielding of the host tissue. Perhaps development of resorbable, tissue-inducing biomaterials and fibroblast-seeded biomaterials will improve the long term biomechanical performance of the reconstructed femur ACL-tibia complex. Carefully planned and executed research studies, in experimental animals and in the clinic, are required to reach this difficult goal.

Cruciate Ligament Reconstruction

Human balance and posture depend on coordinated integration of sensory input from vestibular and visual systems and on somatosensory information from the extremities, trunk, and neck. Dysfunction in any part of the system may result in impaired body balance. The sensory receptors that are found in the muscles, joints, ligaments, tendons, and skin provide input to the central nervous system regarding tissue deformation and force. In recent years there has been strong evidence of a sensory role for the human Anterior Cruciate Ligament (ACL). It may be that the neurophysiologic proprioceptive function of the ACL is as important as its biomechanical role in maintaining joint stability. Hence, there is evidence of a disturbance of sensory input after ACL injury, and several authors have documented a deficit in postural control after ACL injury.

Although mechanical joint stability can be successfully restored after an ACL tear by reconstructive surgery using a free patellar tendon autograft, the ability of ACL reconstruction to restore sensory input is still controversial. Some found evidence of reinnervation in free patellar tendon grafts used for ACL reconstruction in dogs. It has also been reported that knee kinesthesia was restored in midrange of motion after ACL surgery. Barrett postulated that success after ligament reconstruction may not depend directly on the tightness or strength of the reconstruction but rather on the quality of recovery of proprioception.

Regaining neuromuscular control after injury or surgery is a prerequisite for athletes wishing to return to competition.The information about joint and body position and speed and direction of the movement are important factors for maintenance of postural control. Normal proprioceptive feedback provides such information. Functional assessment of the combined peripheral, vestibular, and visual contributions to neuromuscular control is best accomplished through the use of balance and postural sway measurements for the lower extremity.

The patient group, even several years after injury, had impaired postural control in the sagittal plane in single-legged stance on both the injured and the uninjured leg. Twenty-five patients, 8 women and 17 men with a mean age of 27 years (range, 18 to 38), who had undergone unilateral bone-patellar tendon-bone ACL reconstruction (using a middle-third patellar tendon autograft) participated in this study. All patients were recruited from an earlier prospective and randomized study in consecutive order on their agreement to participate. The purpose of that larger study (comprising a total of 45 patients) was to compare the effects of early range of motion training versus immobilization on sagittal knee laxity, thigh muscle strength, range of motion, subjective knee function, and activity level after ACL reconstruction. All of the patients had arthroscopically verified total ACL ruptures and were listed for an ACL reconstruction.The surgery included a medial miniarthrotomy from the tibial tuberosity to 1 cm proximal to the patellar apex.

The patella was not dislocated. The majority of the patients were participating in sports activities when the injury occurred. In addition to the ACL injury, the patients had sustained a total of 20 meniscal injuries and 5 partial medial collateral ligament injuries that did not require surgery. Eighteen of the patients underwent surgery for chronic ACL ruptures, with a mean time from injury to surgery of 81 weeks (range, 14 to 493). Seven of the patients were operated on for acute or subacute ruptures after an average of 8 weeks (range, 2 to 12).

Postoperatively, the patients were randomly allocated for 5 weeks to either immobilization in a plaster cast (12 patients) or to a brace with early range of motion exercises (13 patients). All patients accepted the random allocation to one of the two different postoperative treatments, and both patient groups had equal and supervised rehabilitation. Every patient was prescribed a functional agility program designed to promote the return of proprioception. The mean time elapsed between the surgery and the measurement of postural control was 36 months (range, 27 to 44).

The control group consisted of 20 healthy volunteers, 10 women and 10 men, without any history of significant injuries to the lower limbs or any general disease that might interfere with normal balancing capacity. The mean age was 28 years (range, 17 to 42).

Screening procedure

To rule out any balance disorders, all patients and control subjects underwent a clinical hearing test and an examination of spontaneous, gaze, head shake, and positional nystagmus using the 2D-Video Oculography system before the measurements of postural control. With the subject wearing a specific face mask, the test system records eye movements with an infrared video camera in total darkness. The eye movements are shown on an ordinary video monitor. All patients and control subjects were normal in this respect.

Laxity and scoring

Instrumented measurement of total sagittal knee laxity was performed using the KT-1000 arthrometer. The total anteroposterior tibial displacement was measured with the knee in 30° of flexion using a load level of 135 N. Subjective knee function was evaluated with the Lysholm knee score. The activity level was estimated with the Tegner activity level rating.

Posturography

Postural control in the sagittal and frontal planes was evaluated with dynamic posturography. The test position was with the subject standing on a dual force plate enclosed by a screen, either with the feet parallel and comfortably spaced apart or on one leg at a time. The standardized standing position was with the arms hanging relaxed at the sides, the weightbearing knee in slight flexion (10°), and with the knee of the nonweightbearing leg flexed to 90° while the hip was flexed approximately 45°. The head was held straight, facing forward. Feet were bare and the subjects wore a safety harness to protect them from falling off the platform. To prevent fatigue, a 5-minute break was allowed during the 30-minute standing balance test. The reaction forces between the feet and the ground as well as horizontal anterior-posterior shear forces were recorded by force transducers located in all four quadrants of the dual force plate.

The data were related to the subject's height, thus making it possible to estimate the center of gravity of the swaying body. The posturography measurement was divided in two sections: 1) the sensory organization test and 2) the movement coordination test. The test order between legs was randomized regarding operated/nonoperated in the patient group, and regarding right/left in the control group.

The sensory organization test

The measurement of body sway was done on a fixed force plate in both doublelegged and single-legged stance, with the eyes open and closed. Measurements were also conducted with the force plate sway referenced in a double-legged stance, both with the eyes open and closed. Thus, the sensory organization test consisted of eight separate tests, each including three repeated trials with a duration of 20 seconds. An equilibrium score was used to express the body sway. The score was 100 for no sway, and in case of falling or a sway range of 12.5° or more, the score was defined as 0. The sway range, 12.5°, was based on the theoretical maximum considering the anatomy of the foot, which permits a maximum backward sway of about 4° and a forward sway of about 8°.8 The test procedure was the same as the one described in our previous investigation of postural control in patients with chronic ACL insufficiency.

The movement coordination test

The force plate could also expose the subjects to backward, forward, medial, or lateral translation perturbations. During the medial and lateral perturbations the subjects were standing on a stable support placed on the force plate that made it possible to measure a single-legged stance in the frontal plane. This part was divided into eight separate tests (four on each leg). All the tests were performed in single-legged stance and with the eyes open: three backward translations, three forward translations, three medial translations, and three lateral translations on each leg.

The standard settings of the EquiTest dynamic posturography system were used. The perturbation amplitudes were proportional to body height. The perturbation duration was 300 ms. A sampling frequency of 100 Hz was used. The force reactions to the imposed perturbations were computed and the following parameters describing the response to perturbations were analyzed: 1) the reaction time (in milliseconds) from the onset of force plate motion to the moment when the center of force began to move on the force plate, 2) the time from the beginning of the center of force movement to the point when maximum sway was reached (latency), 3) the amplitude from the baseline of this maximum excursion.

Statistical analysis

For statistical calculations, the mean of the three trials during each sensory organization test was used. The results were evaluated with unpaired or, when appropriate, paired t-tests. A statistical level of P, 0.05 was selected. A multiway analysis of variance was used to evaluate the parameters from the perturbation tests, including the dependence on group (patient's injured leg versus control subject), direction (backward versus forward or medial versus lateral perturbation), and trial number (three tri-als). Tukey's post hoc test was used to analyze the statistical significance between the three trials.

Laxity

The mean total laxity in the ACL-reconstructed knee in the patients treated postoperatively with cast immobilization was 11.5 mm (range, 6 to 15), and in those treated with a brace and early mobilization it was 10.8mm (range, 8 to 13). The difference was not significant (P 5 0.39). Thus, these values were pooled, 11.2 mm (range, 6 to 15), for further analysis. The mean laxity in the patients' uninjured knees was 8.9 mm (range, 6 to 12), thus yielding a mean difference between the reconstructed and uninjured knee of 2.3 mm (range, 22 to 5) (P # 0.001). The mean laxity in the control group was 6.0 mm (range, 5 to

8), which constituted a significant difference compared with the patients' injured knees and with the uninjured knees.

The side-to-side results of the KT-1000 arthrometer tests are summarized in Table 1. In the patient group, the mean difference, laxity of injured minus uninjured knee, was 12 mm (range, -2 to 5). Although the difference in laxity between the reconstructed and uninjured knees for some subjects was rather high, the outcome of the treatment a Negative value indicates larger total anteroposterior displacement in the patient's normal knee. treatment was, as indicated by the scores given below, considered successful. No patients in the operative group had functional giving way. Also, the differences in laxity did not correlate with any of the variables in posturography measurements.

Table 1

The Total Anteroposterior Tibial Displacement in the Patient Group Measured with the KT-1000 Arthrometer

Difference between ACL-reconstructed and normal knee (mm)	*Number of patients* (N=25)
22	1
21	2
0	1
1	1
2	9
3	3
4	7
5	1

Score

The median Lysholm score was 95 (range, 78 to 100) in

the patient group at the time of testing. In the control group, all the subjects had the maximum score of 100. The median Tegner activity level was 7 (range, 3 to 10) in the patient group and 6 (range, 3 to 9) in the control group, which did not constitute any statistical difference.

Posturography

An initial analysis of variance of the posturography results did not show any differences between patients who had undergone postoperative immobilization with plaster and patients who had been subjected to early range of motion rehabilitation in a brace (P values, 0.08 to 0.89), or between patients with a mean side-to-side difference in laxity of less than 3 mm (N 5 14) or 3 mm or more (N = 11) (P values, 0.45 to 0.90). Thus, in the presented results these subgroups were combined.

The sensory organization test on stable support surface: There were no statistically significant differences in the body sway between the patient and control groups when standing on either leg or between the patient's ACL-reconstructed and healthy leg in any of the test situations. The Sensory Organization Test on Sway-Referenced Support Surface. There was a tendency to a greater body sway in the patient group (69.0 6 7.7, mean 6 SD) compared with the control group (90.5 6 2.5) when standing on two legs with the eyes closed, but there was no difference in body sway between the groups when the eyes were open.

Postural reactions to perturbations in the sagittal plane: The reaction time was significantly longer in the patient group than in the control group in both backward and forward perturbations. There was no difference between the patients' ACL-reconstructed and healthy legs. The reaction time was dependent on the number of trials, in that the first exposure yielded greater values than the final one.

The control group had a significantly longer latency in both directions than did the patient group. As regards the influence of direction, latency was significantly shorter in the forward than in the backward direction in both groups. The amplitude of the sway excursion peak, measured in millimeters on an arbitrary scale, was equal for both groups, but lower in forward perturbations. The first trial gave greater amplitudes than did the last one.

Postural reactions to perturbations in the frontal plane: The reaction time did not differ between the groups. However, the reaction time for perturbations in the lateral direction was significantly longer than for those in the medial direction in both groups. The first trial gave significantly longer reaction times than the third one. The latency was significantly longer in the lateral direction, and the first trial gave a longer latency than the third one. No significant difference between the groups or legs was found. The amplitude of the sway caused by the perturbations was significantly larger in the medial than in the lateral direction and for the perturbations in the medial direction during the first trial compared with the last one. No significant differences were found between the patient and control groups or between the injured and uninjured legs.

The static and dynamic standing balance in a patient group at an average of 36 months after ACL reconstruction and compared the results obtained in the injured and the uninjured legs and, in addition, those obtained in a control group. The groups did not differ in age or activity level.

All the patients had postoperatively gone through supervised rehabilitation, training three times every week for 6 to 8 months. Recovery of proprioception and agility training had been the key points in the postoperative rehabilitation.

In the sensory organization test on a stable support surface there was no difference in body sway between the patient and control groups or between the patients' ACL-reconstructed and uninjured legs. In the sensory organization test with a sway-referenced support, double-legged stance, and with the visual system excluded, a tendency to a larger body sway in the patient group. Visual sensory input constitutes a part of the sensorimotor system used in postural control, and its absence thus makes it more difficult to maintain the standing balance on a swayreferenced support.

The indication for surgery after an ACL injury depends on the patient's activity level and on whether instability symptoms are present. Nonoperative treatment is chosen in cases when there are no or only minor instability problems and when a decreased or a modified activity level is acceptable for the patient. Surgery may be chosen later if nonoperative management fails to restore the desired level of function. Rehabilitation after surgery and nonoperative treatment includes training of range of motion, proprioception, and muscle strength, especially for the hamstring muscles.

During the early rehabilitation phase, closed kinetic chain exercises are predominantly used. A successful outcome after any type of treatment regimen implies good functional stability of the injured or reconstructed knee and a return to the patient's former activity level. The methods for assessing the results of treatment have often been limited to measurements of sagittal knee laxity and scoring scales to estimate the functional level. In our investigation, there was no significant difference between the patient subgroups regarding mean total laxity of the reconstructed knee. However, the laxity was significantly higher in the patient's ACL-reconstructed knee than in the uninjured knee or in the control group. Eleven of the 25 patients had a difference in total anteroposterior knee laxity in the injured versus the uninjured knee of 3mm or more.

In spite of this, there was no difference in any of the variables in postural sway between the reconstructed and the uninjured leg or between the patients and the control subjects. It has been found that some patients with an ACL injury can control the sagittal translation of the knee joint during different activities. Success after ACL reconstruction may therefore depend not only on the tightness or strength of the reconstruction but also on the quality of recovery of proprioception. Thus, knee function after an ACL reconstruction should be closely related with knee proprioception. The evaluation of knee surgery and rehabilitation should also include other variables than simply ligament laxity, for example, functional tests of balance and proprioception. Assessment of knee proprioception may be of interest even if measurement of "joint position sense" has not proven sensitive enough to determine a significant difference.

In dynamic balance tests, the first trial of the three translations of the force plate gave larger values in most directions tested. This finding was interpreted as a learning effect or as a neuromuscular adaptation. It was consistent with findings in a previous study where dynamic balance was evaluated in patients with chronic ACL insufficiency.

A significantly poorer first trial during perturbations could also be considered as a risk factor for reinjury. In the sagittal plane, in both the forward and backward directions, there was a significantly longer reaction time observed in the patient group than in the control group for single-legged stance. Further, recorded a shorter latency for the patients than for the control subjects in both directions. The latency was also shorter in forward than in backward perturbations.

On the other hand, the amplitude of the sway excursion peak was equal for both groups, and lower in the forward than in the backward perturbations. These results may indicate that the patients have developed a compensatory proprioceptive mechanism that enhances dynamic knee stability and therefore decreases the latency, especially in forward perturbations. The hamstring muscles are synergistic to the ACL and would also improve the dynamic stability of the ACLdeficient or ACL-reconstructed knee.

In the frontal plane found a significantly larger reaction time and latency in the lateral than in the medial direction for both groups in single-legged stance. The amplitude was larger in the medial direction, in both the patient and the control groups. The ACL prevents medial translation of the tibia in the extended knee but also acts as a secondary restraint to both varus and valgus stresses in all degrees of flexion. However, postural adjustments in the frontal plane are very limited in the knee joint for anatomic reasons. This mechanism gives an opportunity to use larger muscle groups acting directly on the upper segments to move the center of gravity back over the area of support.

Proprioceptive training of the ankle and the hip should thus be considered as an important part in all rehabilitation after an ACL injury and surgery. The purpose of rehabilitation after the ACL surgery is to improve the compensatory mechanisms and restore the pattern for correction.

The average total laxity was significantly larger in the ACL-reconstructed knee than in the uninjured knee or in the control group. In spite of this, there were no differences in any of the test situations in postural sway between the ACL-reconstructed and uninjured leg or between the patients and controls. The differences in laxity of the reconstructed knee did not correlate with any of the posturography variables measured during the perturbations. This supports the hypothesis that rehabilitation, with proprioceptive and agility training, is an important component in restoring the functional stability in the ACL reconstructed knee.

Anterior Cruciate Ligament Injuries

Over the past decade, there has been an increase in interest and participation in sports. Concomitant with this, there has been an increase in sports related injuries, particularly to the lower limbs. Of specifically ligamentous injuries to the knee, rupture of the Anterior Cruciate Ligament (ACL) has been the commonest, and has the greatest potential to cause both short term and long term disability.

Functional Anatomy

The ACL is a broad ligament joining the anterior tibial plateau to the posterior femoral intercondylar notch. The tibial attachment is to a facet, in front of, and lateral to the anterior tibial spine. The femoral attachment is high on the posterior aspect of the lateral wall of the intercondylar notch. It is composed of multiple non-parallel fibers, which, though not anatomically separate, act as three functionally distinct bundles i.e. anteromedial, posterolateral and intermediate. Owing to their wide attachments, variable fiber lengths and the rotation of the ACL that accompanies flexion, the tension in each bundle varies throughout the range of motion. The biomechanical function of the ACL is complex for it provides both mechanical stability and proprioceptive feedback to the knee. In its stabilizing role it has four (main) functions:

— Restrains anterior translation of the tibia;

— Prevents hyperextension of the knee;

— Acts as a secondary stabilizer to valgus stress, reinforcing the medial collateral ligament; and

— Controls rotation of the tibia on the femur in femoral extensions of 0-30°.

This final role is the main clinical function of the ACL. ACL deficiency causes failure of this screw-home mechanism, resulting in subluxation of the tibia on the femur. This critical function in the range of 0 - 30° is important for movements such a side-stepping and pivoting.

Rationale for Treatment

Rupture of the ACL causes significant short term and long term disability. With each episode of ACL instability there is subluxation of the tibia on the femur, causing stretching of the enveloping capsular ligaments and abnormal shear forces on the menisci and on the articular cartilage. Delay in diagnosis and treatment gives rise to increased intra-articular damage as well as stretching of the secondary stabilizing capsular structures. Evidence to support this has been documented by research undertaken in my practice over the past 15 years. In 1976 I studied the relationship of anterior cruciate ligament rupture to meniscal pathology in three groups of patients. The first group comprised 100 consecutive patients who had a primary diagnosis of medial meniscal tear. At surgery 40% of these patients had a ruptured ACL. The next group comprised 100 patients who were operated on primarily for a diagnosis of a lateral meniscal tear. At surgery 60% had a ruptured ACL. The final groups comprised 100 consecutive patients who had tears in both menisci at arthroscopy. It was fascinating that 95% of these patients had a ruptured ACL. Since that time, a number of authors have supported this view that a significant function of the ACL is to protect the menisci and if the ACL is ruptured then meniscal damage will occur. The long-term outlook for an ACL deficient knee is for the development of significant osteoarthrosis. Evidence to support this view has also been documented in my practice.

A series of 100 consecutive total knee replacements demonstrated a 15% incidence of previous ACL rupture. This incidence of ACL rupture is five times higher than that in the general population. Thus it is important to make an early diagnosis of ACL rupture Meniscal injury and long term degenerative damage is to be minimized.

Causes of ACL Rupture

The most common cause of ACL rupture is a traumatic

force being applied to the knee in a twisting moment. This can occur with either a direct or an indirect force. In my practice, about half of the cases of ACL rupture occur without contact, i.e., while side-stepping, pivoting or landing from a jump. The other half are associated with some type of contact, whether it be on the football field, on the snow fields or in a motor vehicle accident. Skiing injuries usually occur during a fall in the inexperienced skier, on hired skis when the bindings do not release.The question arises as to whether there is a predisposition in some people to ACL rupture. A significant number of patients who have sustained bilateral ACL tears. These patients comprise approximately 15% of the total number of patients sustaining rupture of their ACL. Another group of patients, believe, have agenesis of the ACL. In some cases, when have explored the knee within 3 to 4 days of their injury, there is minimal ACL tissue present in the notch. It has been well documented that patients with narrow intercondylar notches are more prone to rupture their ACL's. Their notch is narrow because they have a hypoplastic ACL and hence are more prone to rupture.

Another interesting factor is that patients with recurvatum tend to be more likely to rupture their ACL and are more difficult to treat. I have also noticed a significant number of patients having ruptured their ACL who also have instability of the shoulder. I believe both these groups have a generalized ligamentous disorder.

The classic story of a patient cutting, side-stepping or landing from a jump, and the knee giving way, followed by immediate pain and swelling should alert the diagnostician to the most likely diagnosis of ACL rupture. In my practice a "snap" or "pop" was noted by 60% of the patients. Rapid intra-articular swelling following injury is nearly always due to hemarthrosis. An ACL rupture is present in 75% of patients presenting with an acute hemarthrosis and is due to bleeding from vessels within the torn ligament. Differential diagnoses include osteochondral fracture, peripheral meniscal tear, retinacular tear associated with patella dislocation or subluxation, PCL tear or bleeding disorders.

The diagnosis of ACL tear can be confirmed by three tests: the Lachman test, the dynamic extension test, and the Pivot Jerk test. While the Lachman test and dynamic extension test are helpful in making a diagnosis, particularly in the acute injury, the lateral-pivot jerk test is the most important The lateral pivot jerk test reproduces the rotatory subluxation that occurs in ACL deficiency. The test is difficult to perform and takes residents and fellows in my practice approximately three months of intensive training to be able to adequately perform the jerk test in the unanaesthetised patient. The test is important because the demonstration of the lateral pivot jerk is the replication of the instability that the patient has.

Some authors consider the Lachman test to be the chief confirmation of rupture of the ACL. The ACL commonly heals onto the posterior cruciate ligament producing a falsely negative Lachman test with a fairly firm end point. These patients, however, may still have a positive lateral pivot jerk and clinical instability.

Management of the Ruptured ACL

Once the diagnosis of ruptured ACL is made, management can be divided into conservative and surgical. Correct choice of treatment depends on assessment of three patient factors:

— Age
— Functional disability
— Functional requirements.

A small percentage of the population, perhaps 15%, can survive happily with a ruptured ACL, so a patient profile is important in assessing the indications for surgery. The child, the adolescent, the young adult, the middle aged, and the elderly, represent different surgical problems. Functional disability may vary from an undiagnosed asymptomatic rupture, to the patient whose knee gives way on a daily basis. These differences are due to variations in proprioception muscle control about the knee. Functional requirements vary from sedentary patients with low activity requirements, through those patients with an active social sporting life or physically demanding work, to the elite athlete whose fame and fortune depends upon a highly functional knee. Rupture of the ACL in the child or the elderly is rare and comprises of less than 5% of all ruptured ACLs and are usually treated conservatively.

Rupture in the adolescent is not uncommon and presents its own problems because of skeletal immaturity. Most isometric reconstructions place the growth plate at risk so attempt to treat most of these patients with a conservative program, with proprioceptive rehabilitation and the avoidance of side stepping sports. Reconstruction is delayed to skeletal maturity. However, in elite adolescent athletes with an acute rupture, it is possible to repair their ligament early and to supplement this with a semitendonosis and gracilis reconstruction. It is possible to achieve this acute repair and augmentation while avoiding the growth late by performing the surgery within the epiphyses.

The vast majority of patients, however, fall into the young adult and middle aged groups. Males are more frequently seen than females, though this pattern is reversed in skiers where a disproportionate number of female skiers are injured. The overall type of patient that one sees can be divided into those who definitely need or demand surgery, those who do not want nor warrant surgery, and those patients who require counseling about life style, functional requirements and the expectations of surgery. On one hand there are patients who are not very active, who are not sports minded and who, perhaps, ruptured their ACL on their first skiing holiday. These patients can be recommended a conservative approach.

At the other end of the scale is the athlete at the height of their career who depends on side-stepping activities for their continued economic well-being. The diagnosis having been made, there is little doubt that they should be recommended for early surgery and will be fit to resume full activities within six months. Not everyone is in agreement with this approach, as some athletes feel they would like to try conservative therapy first followed by reconstruction later if necessary. In many sports this may mean that a patient may miss two seasons of professional sport and they may only have 6 or 7 years at the top of their sport. This could therefore account for something like 30% of their playing life whereas if they are operated on urgently they can be back, after rehabilitation, in six months, and therefore only miss one season.

Between these two groups are those people who are keen to participate in community sports such as football, tennis and skiing. With these patients one needs to sit down and discuss the techniques and complications of the procedure, including the costs of the procedure and rehabilitation, the complications and morbidity of the technique, the time and commitment required in the rehabilitation phase and the expected results. A further group requiring special consideration are those patients who present with a chronic ACL rupture with significant osteoarthrosis. They usually present with medial compartment osteoarthrosis following medial meniscectomy and an untreated ACL tear. It is important in these patients to determine and treat their chief complaint. An ACL reconstruction will stabilize the knee but will not result in significant improvement in the arthritic ache. Moreover, as the arthrosis progresses, capsular inflammation will result in significant stiffening of the knee, reducing the clinical instability.

Those patients who present with a chief complaint of arthritic medial compartment ache are best treated by a high tibial osteotomy. Those patients who present with instability as their primary problem will benefit from an ACL reconstruction accompanied with advice that the reconstruction will not significantly improve the medial compartment pain. Those patients who present with both significant instability and pain will benefit from a combined ACL reconstruction followed by high tibial osteotomy.

Surgical Techniques

The development of surgery for ACI instability has been proceeding over the last century. Techniques at the turn of the 20th Century used autograft semitendinosus and gracilis with variable results. Xenografts were employed in Germany in 1912, using Kangaroo tail tendon for ACL substitution. However, results were poor due to problems with infection and graft rejection. It was not until the 1950's when Don O'Donoghue began to aggressively treat knee ligament injuries in American footballers, that a renewed interest in ACL surgery began. Don Slocum from Eugene, Oregon invented the pes plasty in association Bob Larson. This operation was a dynamic tendon transfer attempting to prevent the anterior draw by dynamic muscle contraction. This operation enabled many athletes to return to the sporting arena and that its main function was that it enhanced the proprioceptive control of the knee joint.

With the advent of arthroscopy came renewed research into the anatomy and biomechanics of the normal and injured knee joint. Early anatomical studies finding damage to the lateral capsular ligaments at the time of ACL rupture, caused many of the operative procedures to be aimed at repairing the capsule. Following the failure of repair techniques to ensure stability, focus became centered on substitution-type intra-articular reconstructions. Various graft materials have been tried including autograft, allograft, xenograft and artificial ligaments. Many centers in the world are using allograft patella or Achilles tendon, or allograft anterior cruciate transfers. Artificial ligaments made of fibres such as Dacron or Gortex have also been tried with mixed success. There is an unacceptable failure rate within two years due to either mechanical failure or inflammatory synovitis secondary to breakdown products shed for the graft. A ligament augmentation device has also been widely used. Most studies, however, have not demonstrated that the use of the LAD has any significant advantage over the patella tendon transfer alone.

The use of autograft reconstructions have so far shown the best long term results. The two most common techniques use either the semitendonosis and gracilis, or the middle third of the patella tendon. Currently, my preferred surgical technique for the routine case, is one using an isolated mid-third patella tendon graft placed, and secured arthroscopically. This technique has many advantages over the previous types of surgery. The procedure is relatively non-invasive requiring only small incisions.

The graft can be placed accurately at the isometric points and the fixation of the bone blocks within the femur and tibia with the interference fit screw technique is very secure. This allows early motion and rehabilitation. There is a low perioperative morbidity and a rapid return to the activities of daily living and employment. The operation should be performed in the first week following injury when advantage can be taken of the second phase healing factors. Many authors disagree with this approach, stating that there is an increased rate of arthrofibrosis. It is this second phase healing that causes arthrofibrosis, and that with excellent fixation of the graft and accelerated rehabilitation, this arthrofibrosis factor can be utilized to an advantageous effect towards the graft revascularization and regeneration. It is my practice therefore, to recommend operation within the first week to ten days following injury.

Rehabilitation

Anterior cruciate ligament rehabilitation has undergone considerable changes over the past decade. Intensive research into the biomechanics of the injured and the operated knee have led to a movement away from the techniques of the early 1980's characterized by post operative casting and delayed rehabilitation, to the current early rehabilitation program. The major goals of rehabilitation following ACL surgery are:

— restoration of joint anatomy;

— provision of static and dynamic stability;

— maintenance of the aerobic conditioning and psychological well being; and

— early return to work and sport.

These have required the development of an intensive rehabilitation program in which the patient has to take an active involvement. The graft undergoes physiological changes during its incorporation, as fibroblastic activity changes the biology of the graft to become more ligamentous. The graft is weakest between six and twelve weeks post operatively so programs must be designed to protect the graft during this period.

On the other hand investigations into ligamentous healing have shown that progressive controlled loading provides a stimulus for healing which improves the quality of graft incorporation. More over, early immobilization has advantages such as maintenance of articular cartilage nutrition and retention of bone mineralization. Kinematic research has shown quadriceps contraction causes greatest strain on the anterior cruciate ligament graft between 10° and 45° of flexion.

The anterior cruciate ligament graft lacks the normal mechanoreceptors that provide biofeedback in the uninjured knee. All these factors must be taken into account when designing rehabilitation programs. Our current accelerated rehabilitation program is divided into four phases. In the first one to two weeks the aims of therapy are to decrease pain and swelling, and increase the range of motion of the knee. A post-operative brace is ranged from 30 to 90° and is used until there is adequate quadriceps control. Physiotherapy including CPM is used immediately post operatively. In this early phase there is an emphasis on static contraction of the hamstrings and co-contractions of the hamstrings and the quadriceps. Crutch -walking with partial weight bearing is allowed and the usual modalities are used to reduce pain and swelling.

During the second phase, from two to six weeks, the emphasis is on increasing the range of motion, increasing weight bearing and gaining hamstring and quadriceps control. The patient is usually out of the brace by the third to fourth week. During this phase gait re-education and static proprioception exercises commence. This may include balancing on the affected leg, biofeedback techniques and pool work to maintain conditioning and range of motion. During the third stage, from six to twelve weeks, emphasis is placed on improved muscular control, proprioception and general muscular strengthening. Proprioceptive work progresses from static to dynamic techniques including balance exercises on the wobble board and eventually jogging on a mini-tramp. The patient should have a full range of motion during this stage and gentle resistance work should be added. By the end of this period the patient should be able to cycle normally, swim with a straight leg kick and be able to jog freely on the mini-tramp. The fourth phase of rehabilitation from twelve weeks to six months involves the gradual re-introduction of sports specific exercises aimed at improving agility and reaction times and increasing total leg strength.

Tibial eminence fractures result from extreme ACL tension that causes tibial bone avulsion rather than ACL substance rupture. These fractures functionally disrupt the ACL complex and may cause knee instability. Furthermore, the intraarticular fragment may cause mechanical blocking to knee flexion-extension and joint surface incongruity if the fracture extends into the tibial plateau articular surface. These injuries are most often reported in children, in whom immature growth plates are responsible for the relative bony weakness. These injuries do occur in adults, however, and with significant incidence. Most authors believe that tibial spine fractures are more common in children than in adults, and several studies have reported on tibial eminence fractures in children only.

Biomechanical studies have demonstrated that ligament failure characteristics are influenced by overall age and skeletal maturity. Results of clinical studies have also suggested that the pathologic condition and outcome of tibial eminence fractures are different for skeletally mature patients than they are for those who are skeletally immature. Despite successful healing of the eminence fragment, the ACL may therefore be functionally incompetent, with resulting knee instability. A preferred treatment option may then be ACL reconstruction. Evidence now suggests that the ACL has proprioceptive properties that assist in the neuromuscular control of the knee. Therefore, these properties may be preserved with fixation of tibial eminence fractures. This study was undertaken to evaluate the function of the ACL after the treatment of tibial eminence fractures in skeletally mature patients. The evaluation of ACL function focused on quantitated symptoms, objective knee stability, and knee joint proprioception. For comparison, groups of ACL-deficient and ACL-reconstructed patients were also evaluated.

Ten skeletally mature patients with tibial eminence fractures were treated at our institution during a 5-year period from 1992 to 1997; information about them is summarized in Table 1. The group consisted of five men and five women with an average age of 34.5 years (range, 15 to 66). The mechanism of injury was a noncontact twisting of the knee except in one patient who was a passenger in a motor vehicle accident. All patients developed an acute hemarthrosis at the time of injury. The two patients with type I fractures were treated with closed reduction and immobilization for 4 to 6 weeks in a long leg cast with the knee in full extension.

This was followed by physical therapy to increase range of motion and strengthen the quadriceps muscles. One patient with a type II fracture was treated by closed reduction and immobilization for 4 to 6 weeks followed by physical therapy. One patient with a type III fracture was treated with open reduction and screw fixation similar to the procedure. A 5-cm incision adjacent to the medial aspect of the patellar tendon was created. The fragment was reduced using an awl, and a 4.5-mm cortical screw was placed just anterior to the ACL. Three patients with type III fractures were treated with open reduction and suture fixation. A 5-cm incision was made just medial to the patellar tendon. Two drill holes were made through the anterior tibia and into the reduced fragment adjacent to the ACL insertion.

Nonabsorbable sutures were passed through the drill holes and through the substance of the ACL and then tied over the anterior cortex of the tibia. One patient underwent arthroscopic reduction and suture fixation. An ACL guide was used to reduce the fragment, and drill holes were made through the anterior cortex into the fracture fragment adjacent to the ACL. A nonabsorbable suture was passed through the drill holes and through the ACL arthroscopically, using suture-passing techniques, and then tied over the anterior tibia.

Postoperatively, patients treated with arthroscopic reduction and suture fixation had their knee immobilized for 2 to 3 weeks. Immobilization was followed by physical therapy to increase range of motion and strengthen the quadriceps and hamstring muscles. The average time for patients with displaced eminence fractures to return to their preinjury level of activity, including sports, was 4 months. Two patients with untreated type III fractures were seen more than 1 year after injury with complaints of knee instability. They each had radiographic evidence of tibial spine fracture nonunion, demonstrated by clear separation between the fragment and its bed on the tibia. These patients were evaluated separately from the group whose tibial eminence fractures had been successfully treated.

At follow-up, the Lysholm knee scoring system, which emphasizes knee stability, was used to assess symptoms. Objective laxity was determined by arthrometry, with side-to-side differences obtained with 15, 20, and 30 pounds of force. Proprioception was assessed using three different tests. With the patient standing and blindfolded, the position of the feet was marked on the floor. The patient then raised one leg so that the knee and hip both flexed to 90°. The patient then repositioned his or her foot to the original starting position on the floor as accurately as possible.

The patient practiced the movement twice, then the trial was repeated six times, with measurements taken of the deviation from the original starting position. The contralateral leg was then tested in the same fashion. A supine test was performed with the patient lying on an examination table. The patient's feet were positioned on an adjacent wall approximately 30 cm above his or her hips, keeping the knees and hips flexed 30°. The patient maximally flexed both the hip and knee of the leg being tested and attempted to reposition his or her foot to the original starting position. After two practice movements, the trial was repeated six times with measurements taken of the deviation from the starting position. The contralateral leg was then tested in the same manner.

The patient positioned his or her leg with the knee flexed to 30°, then let the legs hang to 90° and attempted to reposition them to the original starting position of 30° of knee flexion. After two practice movements, a trial of six movements was performed, with measurement of the deviations from the starting point. The contralateral leg was then tested. In all cases, the leg tested first was chosen randomly. For each leg, the six measured deviations were averaged. The difference in average deviation between the legs was then calculated. For comparison with the tibial eminence fracture group and overall validation of the proprioception testing, a control group of 10 patients with known ACL deficiency underwent the three proprioception tests and KT-1000 arthrometer testing. Anterior cruciate ligament deficiency was documented in all cases by MRI. All of the ACLdeficient patients had undergone a period of physical therapy consisting of range of motion and quadriceps and hamstring muscle strengthening before testing.

A third group consisted of 10 patients who had undergone ACL reconstruction with bone-patellar tendon-bone autografts. None of these patients had a pathologic condition of the meniscus or other ligamentous injury, and they experienced no postoperative complications. These patients underwent the three proprioception tests and KT-1000 arthrometer testing. In all cases and for all groups, the examiner was blinded as to which knee had been injured.

The injured knee was compared with the uninjured knee in all three groups using a paired Student's t-test. The Student's t-test was used to compare the tibial eminence fracture group with the ACL-deficient group, the tibial eminence fracture group with the ACL-reconstructed group, and the ACL-reconstructed group with the ACL-deficient group. The Bonferroni adjustment was made to correct for the use of multiple comparisons. Correlation analysis was performed to determine the relationship between knee laxity and proprioception among all patients, using the Spearman nonparametric analysis.

The average Lysholm knee score was 94 for the tibial eminence fracture group. Compared with the ACL-deficient group, the tibial eminence fracture group demonstrated significantly less laxity in all three tests and superior proprioception in all three tests. Compared with the ACL-deficient group, the ACL-reconstruction group demonstrated significantly less laxity in all three tests and superior proprioception in all three tests. The tibial eminence fracture group was not significantly different from the ACL-reconstructed group with respect to laxity and proprioception. When comparing the injured knee with the uninjured knee within the ACL-deficient group, the injured knee had significantly greater laxity and inferior proprioception. Significant differences were not observed when comparing the injured knee with the uninjured knee in the tibial eminence fracture group or the ACL-reconstruction group. The two patients with untreated type III fractures both had greater than a 3-mm side-to-side difference on KT-1000 arthrometer testing, indicating incompetence of the ACL. Furthermore, they had inferior proprioception when compared with the treated tibial eminence fracture group, which was a finding more typical of the ACL deficient group. Correlation was observed between laxity measured by KT-1000 arthrometer testing at 30 pounds of force and proprioception while standing (r 5 0.631), lying supine (r 5 0.582), and sitting (r 5 0.608). One patient experienced loss of range of motion immediately after immobilization of a type I fracture for 6 weeks. Aggressive physical therapy was initiated and full range of motion was regained. No patients demonstrated limited range of motion at follow-up.

The most common treatment recommendation for type I and type II fractures, which are nondisplaced or minimally displaced, has been closed reduction and immobilization. For completely displaced type III fractures, both open and arthroscopic techniques with fixation including sutures, wires, and screws, have been recommended. The goals of treatment include restoring the stabilizing function of the native ACL and eliminating any mechanical block to motion. However, follow-up studies have demonstrated a disturbing amount of residual laxity. Several open surgical techniques have been designed to reduce and stabilize the fragment. Fixation methods have included use of suture, K-wires, and screws. In addition, arthroscopic procedures allow for complete inspection of the joint for associated injuries, including osteochondral injuries and meniscal tears. Furthermore, type II and III fractures may be difficult to differentiate on radiographs and may be more accurately assessed arthroscopically. Arthroscopic techniques for suture fixation and screw fixation. Arthroscopic reduction and fixation may be technically demanding, however. We treated 10 patients with tibial eminence fractures, 8 of whom had acute injuries. Of these, two patients were treated with a closed procedure, five with an open procedure, and one was treated arthroscopically, according to the preference and ability of the treating surgeon.

The eight patients with acute injuries had anatomic reduction and bony union as demonstrated by plain radiographs at follow-up examination. Thus, although the treatment methods differed, the treatment goals of anatomic reduction and bony union were achieved in all cases. Therefore, these patients were used as subjects to analyze ACL function after injury to the ACL complex with bony fracture. Several studies have reported on tibial eminence fractures in children only, and most authors believe that these fractures are more common in children than in adults.

Skeletally mature patients may have different outcomes than children. They do not have the immature growth plates responsible for the relative bony weakness and do not have growth potential that may affect healing and ultimate length of the stretched ACL. In addition, a treatment option for skeletally mature patients with ACL incompetence is ACL reconstruction. Retaining the native ACL by reduction and fixation of the eminence fracture has the potential advantages of maintaining the proprioceptive function and the biomechanical stabilizing function of the ACL.

Biomechanical studies have demonstrated that a significant amount of plastic deformation of the ligament occurs before failure, and clinical reports have demonstrated significant knee laxity at follow-up. Two factors are likely responsible for the residual laxity. One, imperfect reduction may result in malunion that effectively lengthens the ACL complex. Two, plastic deformation of the ligament (by as much as 50%) before ultimate bony fracture may lead to laxity. Several researchers have observed symptoms related to the residual laxity, and others have found patients asymptomatic.

In addition to providing static anterior stability, evidence now suggests that the ACL also acts as a source for neuromuscular control of the knee. Morphologic studies of the ACL have confirmed the presence of mechanoreceptors in and surrounding the human ACL. Differences in proprioception in the ACL-deficient knee when compared with normal control groups have been documented. They demonstrated significantly higher mean values (43.8%) for the injured compared with the uninjured limb in the ACL-deficient group, which was not observed in the control group (4.8%).

When evaluating ACL function, we placed particular emphasis on assessing proprioception in addition to laxity. To validate this new method, we first tested patients with ACL-deficient knees. The ACL-deficient group demonstrated significantly higher mean values for the injured compared with the uninjured limb. The ACL-deficient group showed inferior proprioception in all three proprioception tests when compared with the ACL-reconstructed group and the tibial eminence fracture group. Although our testing method was clearly able to distinguish the ACL-deficient group from both the reconstructed and the tibial eminence fracture groups, it did not show a statistically significant difference between the tibial eminence fracture group and the ACL-reconstructed group. Several factors may contribute to why we did not see a significant difference.

Some studies have demonstrated return of proprioceptive function after ACL reconstruction17 and proprioceptive training. Testing method may not be sensitive sensitive enough to distinguish the more subtle proprioceptive differences between the ACL-reconstructed group and the tibial eminence fracture group. In addition, we found a correlation between knee laxity and proprioception. These results are consistent with the literature demonstrating the proprioceptive function of the ACL. In addition, two patients were seen late with type III eminence fractures, several months after their initial injury. Radiographs revealed nonunion of the bony fragment. In both of these cases, the laxity and proprioception testing results were more typical of the ACL-deficient patients.

The standing method of testing, however, requires the proprioception of the contralateral hip and knee in addition to the ipsilateral hip for foot placement on the floor. We developed the supine and sitting tests in an effort to minimize the contribution of hip and contralateral knee proprioception to the overall measurements. With the patient in the supine position, the involvement of the contralateral hip and knee is eliminated when positioning the foot, although the ipsilateral hip participates. With the patient in the seated position, involvement of both hips and the contralateral knee are eliminated when positioning the foot.

In addition, the knee flexion angle for the supine and seated position is 30°, which is similar to that of a Lachman examination. Also, the force acting on the tibia due to gravity in both the supine and seated examinations has a greater anterior-posterior component than in the standing position, and thus may better isolate ACL proprioception. We have demonstrated that proper treatment of tibial eminence fractures in adults restores both stability and proprioception to the knee. Thus, reduction and fixation of the fracture fragment, either open or arthroscopic, is a viable alternative to ACL reconstruction in adult patients with tibial eminence fractures. Rehabilitation time is not significantly different because bone-to-bone healing is still required; however, there is no graft site morbidity or problems related to allograft tissue. Therefore, tibial eminence fractures in adults, often treated with ACL reconstruction, can also be treated successfully with fracture reduction and fixation, yielding a functionally stable knee that retains its proprioceptive function.

Future Directions

The 'tissue engineering' approach to ACL reconstruction uses resorbable scaffolds consisting of tissue-derived and/ or synthetic materials to induce neoligament formation. This concept was originally developed for repair of other connective tissues including skin, bone, and cartilage. In contrast to permanent synthetic prostheses that lose strength with time, the mechanical behavior of these implants should improve with time due to neoligament tissue development and remodeling. Fibroblast-seeding of resorbable scaffolding devices is another promising concept that is currently a focus of ACL reconstruction research in our laboratories at Robert Wood Johnson Medical School.

Although the use of resorbable synthetic polymers for tendon/ligament reconstruction is an interesting idea, few reports are found. A resorbable device composed of braided polyglycolic acid suture (Dexon) was successfully used to reinforce ACL repair in dogs. Others reconstructed the rabbit Achilles tendon with resorbable fibers composed of dimethyltrimethylene carbonate and trimethylene carbonate. At 26 weeks, the implanted fibers were still intact, and fibrous tissue in the center of the prosthesis was disorganized. A more rapid fiber degradation rate is needed to promote earlier tensile loading and organization of the host ingrowth tissue.

In addition to synthetic polymers, tissue-derived materials also show promise for development of novel ACL reconstruction devices. Type I collagen is the major structural component of tendons and ligaments. It can be extracted from tissues and processed into thin, high-strength fibers to make resorbable scaffolds with in vivo mechanical behavior similar to autografts.

The resorption rate of collagen can be controlled by the extent of crosslinking, and no permanent wear debris is generated during its resorption. Collagen is not highly antigenic, and is chemotactic for fibroblasts and other cells involved in tissue repair. Reconstituted collagen has been used extensively as a scaffold to accelerate dermal repair. Growth factors and other extracellular matrix components can be added to enhance the biological activity of collagen.

Surgically reconstructed both the rabbit Achilles tendon and ACL using collagen fiber-based scaffolds. These degradable implants induce deposition of neotendon and neoligament tissue. The collagen scaffolds experience early strength loss, followed by tissue ingrowth and strength regain, similar to autogenous grafts. The rate of strength regain in neotendon and neoligament tissue is proportional to the degradation rate of the implanted collagen scaffold. In surgical bone tunnels, the collagen scaffolds resorb rapidly, and induce rapid ingrowth of fibrous tissue and bone. These results suggest that tissue ingrowth in the bone tunnels might provide biological fixation for collagen prostheses used for ACL reconstruction.

7

Sports Injuries

Low Back Injury

Low back injuries in athletes are among the most challenging and frustrating clinical situations for sports physicians to diagnose and treat. Low back injuries account for 10% to 15% of all athletic injuries and most frequently involve the soft tissue surrounding the spine. Under these circumstances, conventional diagnostic imaging such as radiographs, CT scans, and MRI are frequently equivocal in diagnosing these injuries. There are no standard clinical tests for documenting the extent of soft tissue damage. Such tests could assist the physician with the choice of treatments. There is no consensus with regard to a treatment regimen for low back injury in terms of the rest duration, the specific rehabilitation protocol, or the criteria for return of athletes to training and competition. Identification of the risk factors that predispose an athlete to sustain a low back injury would provide valuable assistance to the clinician in the selection of preventive or rehabilitation treatment strategies, given the lack of standard diagnostic tools.

Many of the etiologic factors associated with low back injury are mechanical in nature and result from sudden movements that impose sudden loading to the spine. The neuromuscular control system must respond to the external trunk loading with compensatory muscle forces necessary to mechanically stabilize the lumbar spine. Therefore, muscle control of lumbar spine stability is an important factor in determining trunk kinematic response to sudden loading and the subsequent likelihood of injury. However, because of the spine's multiple degrees of freedom, the motor control for stabilizing it is extremely complex. If the motor control of the lumbar spine is deficient or impaired, it may lead to low back injury, particularly under sudden loading conditions.

Deficiencies in motor control of the lumbar spine have been proposed as one of the possible mechanisms predisposing people to acute low back injury. Athletes, despite an apparent clinical recovery from an acute low back injury, exhibit prolonged trunk muscle response time when confronted with sudden loading in comparison with athletes with no history of low back injury. Similar altered neuromuscular recruitment patterns and impaired proprioception have been reported in athletes with ACL-deficient knees, ankle sprains, shoulder dislocations, and generalized joint laxity.

Several prospective studies have documented a decrease in recurrent ankle and knee injuries after a specific rehabilitation program emphasizing motor control and proprioception training. A number of biomechanical, psychosocial, and demographic risk factors for sustaining an acute low back injury have been identified in the general population. Job dissatisfaction and a history of previous or current low back injury are among the best known risk factors. However, to the best of our knowledge, there are no similar prospective studies of athletes. If there are risk factors that predispose athletes to sustain a low back injury, the athlete is at risk of recurrent or chronic problems unless those risk factors are identified and the appropriate rehabilitation and preventive measures are taken. Therefore, the purpose of this prospective study was to investigate whether a history of low back injury and dissatisfaction with the coach and teammates could predict the low back injury occurrence among varsity athletes during a 1-year period. The null hypothesis was that the likelihood of sustaining a low back injury is uniformly distributed among all athletes in the population studied.

Materials and Methods

A total of 679 Yale University varsity athletes representing 30 sport disciplines were surveyed, including 422 men and 257 women with an average age of 19 years (SD, 1) (see Table 3). The athletes completed a 16-item questionnaire at the time of their medical examination at the beginning of the 1999/2000 season. The athletes were assured that their responses would be confidential and that the information provided would be used for research purposes only.

The survey was reviewed and approved by the Medical Director of Yale University Athletics and the Human Investigation Committee. In addition to the demographic characteristics (sex, age, height, weight, and sport), the questionnaire examined psychosocial factors (satisfaction with coaches and teammates) and history of past low back injury. The athletes were free to interpret their definition of satisfaction with coaches and teammates and then assign it to the numeric scale provided in the questionnaire. To determine the athletes' history of low back injury, we asked whether they had sustained a low back injury within the last 5 years, when the low back injury occurred, how long symptoms persisted, how much time was lost from regular training, and whether there was a family history of low back pain or low back injury.

The athletes were observed for 1 year, and the low back injuries sustained during that time interval were documented. For the purpose of this study, an injury was defined as any low back pain that caused an athlete to miss or not participate fully in at least three practice sessions or competitions and that resulted in a visit to a sports physician. Injured athletes were identified as a result of their visit to the sports clinic.

Multiple binary logistic regression analysis was performed to identify risk factors that would best predict occurrence of low back injury among the athletes. The incidence of low back injury and relative risks were also computed with respect to the factors gathered from the questionnaire.

$$\text{Relative risk} = \frac{\text{Incidence of low back injury in exposed group}}{\text{Incidence of low back injury in unexposed group}}$$

where the exposed group is athletes with a history of a low back injury within the last 5 years and the unexposed group is athletes without a history of low back injury.

$$\text{Incidence} = \frac{\text{Number of new low back injury cases}}{\text{Number of athletes}}$$

Data analysis was performed for all sports combined as well as for noncontact and contact sports separately. Ice hockey, football, and lacrosse represented the contact sports because direct player contact is permitted by the rules of these sports. When appropriate, a two-proportions test (Minitab) was used to examine whether there were significant differences between contact and noncontact sports.

Of the 679 athletes surveyed, 124 (18.3%) reported that they had a history of a low back injury within the past 5 years, and almost 90% of these cases were sportsrelated (Tables 1 and 2). There was no difference in injury rates between men and women or between contact and noncontact sports. However, athletes participating in contact sports had a significantly higher percentage of injuries caused by contact with another player or by impact than did athletes who participated in noncontact sports (20.9% versus 2.9%, Table 1). The majority of the reported sports-related back injuries within the past 5 years were caused by selfinitiated actions (90.1%, Table 1).

Twenty-two percent of the athletes (155) failed to respond to the question with regard to satisfaction with coaches, and 17% (118) did not respond to the question on satisfaction with teammates. Among those who responded, fewer than 5% reported that they were dissatisfied or somewhat dissatisfied with their coaches or their teammates. However, there was no significant association between nonresponse and low back injury during the follow-up period.

Overall, 6.8% of the surveyed athletes sustained a low back injury in the following season/year (Tables 1 and 2). Of these injuries, 26% (12) were serious, and the athletes were placed on disability, which meant that they were not allowed to practice or play at all. There was no significant difference in this respect between contact and noncontact sports or between men and women (Table 1).

Multiple, stepwise, binary, logistic regression analysis returned the factor "currently have low back pain" as the single best predictor for sustaining a low back injury in the following season. Other significant single predictors of low back injury were a history of low back injury within the last 5 years, how long ago the low back injury occurred, how many days were missed from training because of the low back injury, and how long it took to return to regular training and competition (Table 3). However, all of the factors mentioned were highly correlated and none of their combinations improved the overall prediction for sustaining a low back injury in the following season. None of the psychosocial (satisfaction with coach and teammates) or demographic items (age, sex, sport) were significant as a predictor or a factor in the regression model. The severity of injury (placed on disability or not) was poorly predicted by this model.

Athletes who had low back pain at the time of the survey were six times more likely to sustain a low back injury in the following season/year than athletes without a history of low back injury (Table 3). A history of low back injury at any time within the last 5 years indicated a three times greater risk for sustaining a future low back injury.

There was no difference in relative risks for these two factors between contact and noncontact sports. However,

Table 1

Low Back Injury Rates and Causes among Yale Varsity Athletes

Variable	All sports		Contact sportsa		Noncontact sports	
	N	(%)	N	(%)	N	(%)
Total number of athletes surveyed	679		217		462	
Injured during the following (99/00) season	46	(6.8)	20	(9.2)	26	(5.6)
History of low back injury within the last 5 years	124	(18.3)	48	(22.1)	76	(16.5)
Not sports-related (accidents)	2	(1.6)	0	(0.0)	2	(2.6)
No specific cause	11	(8.9)	5	(10.4)	6	(7.9)
Sports-related	111	(89.5)	43	(89.6)	68	(89.5)
Injury resulted from contact/impact	11	(9.9)	9	(20.9)	2	(2.9)
Injury resulted from self-initiated action	100	(90.1)	34	(79.1)	66	(97.1)
Change of direction	11	(11.0)	2	(5.9)	9	(13.6)
Erging/rowing	5	(5.0)	0	(0.0)	5	(7.6)
Jumping	4	(4.0)	1	(2.9)	3	(4.6)
Overuse	3	(3.0)	0	(0.0)	3	(4.5)
Running	9	(9.0)	4	(11.9)	5	(7.6)
Sudden stops	2	(2.0)	0	(0.0)	2	(3.0)
Throwing	6	(6.0)	2	(5.9)	4	(6.1)
Weight training/lifting	36	(36.0)	21	(61.8)	15	(22.7)
Diving	2	(2.0)	0	(0.0)	2	(3.0)
Other	8	(8.0)	1	(2.9)	7	(10.6)
Multiple causes	14	(14.0)	3	(8.8)	11	(16.7)

when a family history of low back pain or injury was evaluated independently of present low back pain or a history of low back injury within the last 5 years, a two times greater risk was found between contact and noncontact sports (Table 3). When a history of low back injury within the last 5 years was combined with a family history of low back pain or injury, the relative risks for all sports,

We found that a history of low back injury within the past 5 years and related factors (how long ago low back injury occurred, whether low back pain was currently present, time missed from training, time back to regular training/ competition) were significant predictors for sustaining a low back injury in the following athletic season. Of these related factors, the presence of low back pain at the beginning of the season indicated a six-fold increase in the risk for sustaining a low back injury in the following year. Bigos et al.1 reached an almost identical conclusion from their prospective study of 3020 aircraft employees. They found that current or recent back problems combined with work dissatisfaction were the most predictive factors for reporting acute back pain at work during a 4-year follow-up period. The presence of low back pain at baseline was also the most significant risk factor for reinjury among nursing students and army airborne soldiers. In contrast to the data from those populations, no psychosocial or demographic factors were found to be significant predictors for low back injury in our study, most likely because athletes are highly motivated and satisfied with their sport activities. Moreover, they have fewer financial and social incentives to exaggerate or to pretend to suffer from a low back injury. Collegiate athletes are otherwise healthy and

Table 3

Results of a Multiple Logistic Regression for Predicting Future Low Back Injuries among Athletes and the Relative Risks Computed for Single Binary Predictors

Regression model	*Significance as a single predictor of low back injury (P value)*	*Relative risk*		
		All sports	*Contact sports*	*Non-contact sports*
Family history of low back injury or pain	0.091	1.7	2.5	1.1
History of injury within the last 5 years	0.000	3.1	3.5	2.7
Family history and injury within the last 5 years		4.1	7.1	2.6
How long ago did injury occur	0.000			
Currently have low back pain	0.000	6.5	5.6	6.5
Days missed from training	0.000			
Time back to regular training/competition	0.000			
Satisfaction with coach	0.704			
Satisfaction with teammates	0.985			

Table 2

Low Back Injury Rates among Yale Varsity Athletes by Sport[a]

Sport	*Surveyed*	*Injured during 1999/2000 season*		*History of low back injury within last 5 years*	
		N	(%)	N	(%)
Baseball-M	28	0	(0.0)	4	(14.3)
Basketball-M	19	6	(31.6)	6	(31.6)
Basketball-W	14	0	(0.0)	3	(21.4)
Crew-M	60	3	(5.0)	12	(20.0)
Crew-W	31	2	(6.5)	4	(12.9)
Cross country-M	15	1	(6.7)	0	(0.0)
Cross country-W	24	0	(0.0)	2	(8.3)
Diving-W	3	0	(0.0)	3	(100.0)
Fencing-M	14	0	(0.0)	0	(0.0)
Fencing-W	17	1	(5.9)	3	(17.6)
Field hockey-W	23	0	(0.0)	3	(13.0)
Football-M	112	13	(11.6)	30	(26.8)
Golf-M	22	0	(0.0)	4	(18.2)
Golf-W	9	1	(11.1)	2	(22.2)

Gymnastics-W	11	1	(9.1)	4	(36.4)
Ice hockey-M	29	5	(17.2)	4	(13.8)
Ice hockey-W	18	2	(11.1)	2	(11.1)
Lacrosse-M	30	0	(0.0)	8	(26.7)
Lacrosse-W	30	0	(0.0)	4	(13.3)
Soccer-M	29	3	(10.3)	5	(17.2)
Soccer-W	21	1	(4.8)	1	(4.8)
Softball-W	7	0	(0.0)	1	(14.3)
Swimming-M	35	0	(0.0)	1	(2.9)
Swimming-W	23	3	(13.0)	3	(13.0)
Tennis-M	16	0	(0.0)	2	(12.5)
Tennis-W	10	2	(20.0)	4	(40.0)
Track-M	39	3	(7.7)	6	(15.4)
Track-W	23	0	(0.0)	3	(13.0)
Volleyball-W	27	2	(7.4)	6	(22.2)
Not specified	3	0	(0.0)	0	(0.0)

constitute a homogeneous group with regard to their age and fitness level.

The main limitation of our approach was that we studied varsity athletes from only one institution. However, the low back injury rate from our study (6.8%) correlates with the findings of Keene et al.,18 who reported an injury rate of 7 per 100 participants for collegiate athletes. They reviewed records of 4790 athletes who competed in 17 varsity sports over a 10-year period. Therefore, athletes in the present study were representative of the intercollegiate population, and our findings can be extrapolated with a high level of confidence.

No attempt was made in our study to express the low back injury incidence relative to the exposure time during practice or competition (player hours) for several reasons. First, we were not comparing the injury incidence among the sport disciplines or between sexes, for which such a normalization of data would be necessary.19 Second, the rationale for our hypothesis was that if some risk factors exist that predispose an athlete to sustain a low back injury, then a previous low back injury is a good predictor for future injuries. For this purpose, we documented any low back injury sustained by an athlete regardless of whether the injury was sustained during competition, practice, or leisure activity. If this hypothesis were true, even athletes who are not starters would still be susceptible to low back injury during any other physical activity. On the basis of our results, the null hypothesis that the likelihood of sustaining low back injury is uniformly distributed among all athletes in the population should be rejected.

The finding that only a history of previous low back injury predicted the occurrence of another low back injury in the following year suggests that biomechanical, motor control, or other risk factors predispose an athlete to sustain recurrent back injuries. In another study, we documented delayed trunk muscle responses to sudden loading in athletes after they had clinically recovered from an acute low back injury and returned to competition. This documented motor control impairment may be one of the important risk factors. Our observation that over 90% of low back injuries sustained within the previous 5 years occurred due to self-initiated actions is also consistent with the hypothesis that impaired motor control may be a significant risk factor.

Similar hypotheses involving motor control impairment correlation with injury risks have been formulated in research on the ankle, knee, and shoulder joints. Several reports suggest that motor control impairment could be improved with specific therapy focused on motor control and proprioception training. Perhaps similar preventive and rehabilitative strategies could be employed for athletes with low back injury. A low back rehabilitation program that focuses on motor control and is used even after full clinical recovery and return to competition may prevent the recurrence of low back injury in young athletes. Future studies should address these issues.

Regardless of the cause of the recurrent back injury, the more immediate application of our results is the message to sports clinicians and trainers that athletes with a history of low back injury have a three to six times greater risk of sustaining a recurrent injury than athletes without such a history. This risk factor should be taken into consideration for preseason sports screening as well as for possible design of preventive exercises during practice.

Childhood Sports Injuries

Childhood sports injuries may be inevitable, but there are some things you can do to help prevent them:

— Enroll your child in organized sports through schools, community clubs, and recreation areas where there may be adults who are certified athletic trainers (ATC). An ATC is also trained in the prevention, recognition and immediate care of athletic injuries.

— Make sure your child uses the proper protective gear for a particular sport. This may lessen the chances of being injured.

— Warmup exercises, such as stretching and light jogging, can help minimize the chance of muscle strain or other soft tissue injury during sports. Warmup exercises make the body's tissues warmer and more flexible. Cooling down exercises loosen the body's muscles that have tightened during exercise.2 Make warmups and cool downs part of your child's routine before and after sports participation.

And don't forget to include sunscreen and a hat (where possible) to reduce the chance of sunburn, which is actually an injury to the skin. Sun protection may also decrease the chances of malignant melanoma-a potentially deadly skin cancer-or other skin cancers that can occur later in life. It is also very important that your child has access to water or a sports drink to stay properly hydrated while playing.

Treat Injuries with "RICE"

If your child receives a soft tissue injury, commonly known

as a sprain or a strain, or a bone injury, the best immediate treatment is easy to remember.

Rice (Rest, Ice, Compression, and Elevation) the injury. Get professional treatment if any injury is severe. A severe injury means having an obvious fracture or dislocation of a joint, prolonged swelling, or prolonged or severe pain.

— *Rest:* Reduce or stop using the injured area for 48 hours. If you have a leg injury, you may need to stay off of it completely.

— *Ice:* Put an ice pack on the injured area for 20 minutes at a time, 4 to 8 times per day. Use a cold pack, ice bag, or a plastic bag filled with crushed ice that has been wrapped in a towel.

— *Compression:* Compression of an injured ankle, knee, or wrist may help reduce the swelling. These include bandages such as elastic wraps, special boots, air casts and splints. Ask your doctor which one is best.

— *Elevation:* Keep the injured area elevated above the level of the heart. Use a pillow to help elevate an injured limb.

Sprains and Strains

A sprain is an injury to a ligament-a stretching or a tearing. One or more ligaments can be injured during a sprain. A ligament is a band of tough, fibrous tissue that connects two or more bones at a joint and prevents excessive movement of the joint. Ankle sprains are the most common injury in the United States and often occur during sports or recreational activities. Approximately 1 million ankle injuries occur each year and 85 percent of these are sprains. A strain is an injury to either a muscle or a tendon. A muscle is a tissue composed of bundles of specialized cells that, when stimulated by nerve impulses, contract and produce movement. A tendon is a tough, fibrous cord of tissue that connects muscle to bone.

Growth Plate Injuries

In some sports accidents and injuries, the growth plate may be injured. The growth plate is the area of developing tissues at the end of the long bones in growing children and adolescents. When growth is complete, sometime during adolescence, the growth plate is replaced by solid bone. The long bones in the body are the long bones of the fingers, the outer bone of the forearm, the collarbone, the hip, the bone of the upper leg, the lower leg bones, the ankle, and the foot. If any of these areas become injured, seek professional help from a doctor who specializes in bone injuries in children and adolescents (pediatric orthopaedist).

Repetitive Motion Injuries

Painful injuries such as stress fractures (where the ligament pulls off small pieces of bone) and tendinitis (inflammation of a tendon) can occur from overuse of muscles and tendons. These injuries don't always show up on x-rays, but they do cause pain and discomfort. The injured area usually responds to rest. Other treatments include *rice*, crutches, cast immobilization, or physical therapy.

Playing rigorous sports in the heat requires close monitoring of both body and weather conditions. Heat injuries are always dangerous and can be fatal. Children perspire less than adults and require a higher core body temperature to trigger sweating. Heat-related illnesses include dehydration (deficit in body fluids), heat exhaustion (nausea, dizziness, weakness, headache, pale and moist skin, heavy perspiration, normal or low body temperature, weak pulse, dilated pupils, disorientation, fainting spells), and heat stroke (headache, dizziness, confusion, and hot dry skin, possibly leading to vascular collapse, coma, and death). These injuries can be prevented.

Playing safe in the heat is cool

— Recognize the dangers of playing in the heat.

— Respond quickly if heat-related injuries occur.

— Schedule regular fluid breaks during practice and games.

— Drinking water is the best choice; others include fruit juices and sports drinks.

— Kids need to drink 8 ounces of fluid every 20 minutes, plus more after playing.

— Make player substitutions more frequently in the heat.

— Wear light-colored, "breathable" clothing, and wide-brimmed hats

— Use misting water sprays on the body to keep cool.

Exercise is beneficial

Even though Raoul got hurt, his involvement in sports is important. Exercise may reduce his chances of obesity, which is becoming more common in children. It may also lessen his risk of diabetes, a disease that is sometimes associated with a lack of exercise and poor eating habits. As a parent, it is important for you to match your children to the sport, and not push him or her too hard into an activity that he or she may not like or be capable of doing. Sports also helps children build social skills and provides them with a general sense of well-being. Sports participation is an important part of learning how to build team skills.

Football

This popular sport "leads the pack" in the number of injuries, especially in boys, in organized sports. Common injuries and locations: Bruises, sprains, strains, pulled muscles, soft tissue tears such as ligaments, broken bones, internal injures (bruised or damaged organs), back injuries, sunburn. Knees and ankles are the most common injury sites.

Safest playing with: Helmet; mouth guard; shoulder pads; athletic supporters for males; chest/rib pads; forearm, elbow, and thigh pads; shin guards; proper shoes; sunscreen; water.

Prevention: Proper use of safety equipment, warm-up exercises, proper coaching and conditioning.

Basketball

This popular sport has the highest rate of knee injuries requiring surgery among girls. Common injuries and locations: Sprains, strains, bruises, fractures, scrapes, dislocation, cuts, dental injuries. Ankles, knees, (injury rates are higher in girls, especially for the anterior cruciate ligament, the wide ligament that limits rotation and forward movement of the shin bone), shoulder (rotator cuff strains and tears, where tendons at the end of muscles attach to the upper arm and shoulder bones). Safest playing with: Eye protection, elbow and knee pads, mouth guard, athletic supporters for males, proper shoes, water. If playing outdoors, add a hat and sunscreen.

Prevention: Strength training (particularly knees and shoulders), aerobics (exercises that develop the strength and endurance of heart and lungs), warmup exercises, proper coaching, and use of safety equipment.

Soccer

This sport has dramatically increased in popularity in the past two decades in the U.S.

Common injuries: Bruises, cuts and scrapes, headaches, sunburn. Safest playing with: Shin guards, athletic supporters for males, cleats, sunscreen, water.

Prevention: Aerobic conditioning and warmups, and proper training in "heading" the ball. ("Heading" is using the head to strike or make a play with the ball.)

Baseball and Softball

Sometimes called "America's favorite pastime."

Common injuries: Soft tissue strains, impact injuries that include fractures due to sliding and being hit by a ball, sunburn.

Safest playing with: Batting helmet, shin guards, elbow guards, athletic supporters for males, mouth guard, sunscreen, cleats, hat, breakaway bases.

Prevention: Proper conditioning and warmups.

Gymnastics

The performance of systematic exercises.

Common injuries: Sprains and strains of soft tissues. Safest playing with: Athletic supporters for males, safety harness, joint supports (such as neoprene wraps), water.

Prevention: Proper conditioning and warmups.

Track and Field

Competing at running, walking, jumping, throwing, or pushing events.

Common injuries: Strains, sprains, scrapes from falls.

Safest playing with: Proper shoes, athletic supporters for males, sunscreen, water.

Prevention: Proper conditioning and coaching.

How your child can prevent sports injuries

— Be in proper physical condition to play the sport. Know and abide by the rules of the sport.

— Wear appropriate protective gear (for example, shin guards for soccer, a hard-shell helmet when facing a baseball or softball pitcher, a helmet and body padding for ice hockey).

— Know how to use athletic equipment.
— Always warm up before playing.
— Avoid playing when very tired or in pain.
— Get a preseason physical examination.
— Make sure there is adequate water orother liquids to maintain proper hydration.

Ankle Acute Injuries

Ligamentous injuries around the ankle joint are among the most common sporting injuries especially in jumping sports (e.g., basketball, volleyball). They are not always well managed. Associated injuries are frequently not diagnosed and the rehabilitation of ligamentous injuries is often inadequate leading to a high rate of recurrence.

The ankle contains three joints. The talocrural or ankle joint is a hinge joint formed between the inferior surface of the tibia and the superior surface of the talus. The medial and lateral malleoli provide additional articulations and stability to the ankle joint. The movements at the ankle joint are plantarflexion and dorsiflexion. The inferior tibiofibular joint the articulation of the distal parts of the fibula and tibia. The inferior tibiofibular joint is supported by the tibiofibular ligaments or syndesmosis. A small amount of rotation is present at this joint. The subtalar joint between the talus and calcaneus is divided into an anterior and posterior articulation separated by the sinus tarsi. The main roles of the subtalar joint are to provide shock absorption, to permit the foot to adjust to uneven ground and to allow the foot to remain flat on the ground when the leg is at an angle to the surface.

The lateral ligament consists of three parts: the anterior talofibular ligament (ATFL) which passes as a flat band from the tip of the fibula anteriorly to the lateral talar neck; the calcaneofibular ligament (CFL), which is a cord-like structure directed somewhat posteriorly; and the posterior talofibular ligament (PTFL), which runs posteriorly from the fibula to the talus. The medial or deltoid ligament of the ankle is a strong, fan shaped ligament extending from the medial malleolus anteriorly to the navicular and talus, inferiorly to the calcaneus and posteriorly to the talus.

Inversion injuries are far more common than eversion injuries due to the relative instability of the lateral joint and weakness of the lateral ligaments compared to the medial ligament. Eversion injuries are seen occasionally. The strong medial ligament requires a greater force to be injured, therefore, these sprains usually take longer to rehabilitate. Ankle injuries are listed in Table 4.

Table 4: Ankle acute injuries.

Common

- Ligament Sprain
    - lateral ligaments

Less Common

- Ligament Injuries
    - medial ligament
- AITFL sprain
- Peroneal Dislocation
- Fractures
    - lateral / medial / posterior malleolus
    - tibial plafond

—base of the 5th metatarsal

—anterior process of calcaneus

—lateral process of talus

—os trigonum

— Dislocated Ankle (fracture/dislocation)

— Tendon Rupture

— tibialis posterior

— peroneal tendons

Uncommon but not to be Missed

— Reflex Sympathetic Dystrophy (post surgery)

— Greenstick or Growth Plate Fractures (children)

— Ruptured Syndesmosis

The most important component of the assessment of ligamentous injuries is to determine the degree, if any, of instability present in the joint. This will determine the management of the injury. A comprehensive rehabilitation program is required in athletes with ligamentous injuries of the ankle if they are to return to their sport with full functional capacity and avoid recurrence of the injury. Occasionally, other structures are damaged in addition to the ligaments. If these are not recognized and treated, prolonged pain and disability may result. These include fractures around the ankle joint, osteochondral fractures of the dome of the talus and dislocation of the peroneal tendons.

The mechanism of onset is an important clue to the diagnosis. An inversion injury suggests lateral ligament damage, an eversion injury medial ligament damage. The presence of a compressive component indicates the possibility of osteochondral injury. At the time of the injury, the athlete may have heard a snap or tear. Unlike the significance of a 'snap' or 'pop' in an acute knee injury, this sensation is not of diagnostic significance The location of pain will give an indication as to the ligaments injured. The most common site is over the anterolateral aspect of the ankle involving the ATFL. Occasionally in severe injuries, both medial and lateral ligamentous structures will be damaged. Most ankle joint injuries are accompanied by swelling. The site of the swelling may give an indication of the location of the pathology, but the degree of swelling is usually, but not always a reliable indication of severity. The degree of disability, both immediately following the injury and subsequently, is an important indicator of the severity of the injury. The initial management, the use of the *rice* regimen and the duration of restricted weight bearing after the injury should all be noted. A previous history of ankle injury and an assessment of the quality of the post-injury rehabilitation programme should be obtained. Subsequent use of protective tape and braces should be noted.

Examination of the ankle requires assessment of the degree of instability present and the grading of the ligamentous injury. Examination should detect functional disability such as loss of range of motion, reduced strength and reduced proprioception.

Investigations

X-ray including A-P, lateral and at least one oblique view should be performed after ankle sprains in situations where instability is present or when acute bony tenderness is present on the malleoli or the medial or lateral dome of the talus. X rays of the ankle joint must include the base of the 5th metatarsal to exclude associated fracture. An osteochondral fracture may not be apparent on initial X-ray. If significant pain and disability are present despite appropriate treatment 4 - 6 weeks after an apparent 'routine' ankle sprain, specialist sports physician or orthopedic surgeon referral is indicated. A radioisotopic bone scan may be performed to exclude an osteochondral fracture.

Lateral Ligament Injuries

Lateral ligament injuries occur in activities involving rapid changes in direction, especially on uneven surfaces. They are also seen when contact with another competitor's feet causes imbalance in jumping or landing. They are one of the most common injuries seen in basketball, volleyball, netball and most football codes. In the typical inversion and plantarflexion injury, the three parts of the lateral ligament are usually damaged in order depending on the severity of the sprain.

The ATFL is the first ligament damaged, followed by the CFL and finally the PTFL. Complete tear of all three ligaments results in a dislocation of the ankle joint and is frequently associated with a fracture. In the assessment of lateral ligament injuries, each of the three components of the ligament must be examined and the overall degree of instability determined. Lateral ligament injuries are divided into three grades. Grade I corresponds to a minor tear with pain produced by stressing the ligament, but no laxity. Grade II injuries are painful on stressing the ligament and show some degree of laxity on examination, but have a firm end point. Grade III injuries show gross laxity without a discernible endpoint. Grading of these injuries gives a guide to prognosis and helps determine the rate of rehabilitation. The usual mechanism of lateral ligament injury is inversion and plantarflexion. This may be accompanied by an audible snap, crack or tear. Depending on the severity of the injury, the athlete may have been able to continue activity immediately or have been forced to rest. Swelling usually appears soon after the injury, although occasionally it may be delayed some hours.

Treatment of lateral ligament injuries

The management of lateral ligament injuries of all three grades follows the same principles.

Initial management

The initial management of lateral ligament injuries requires the *rice* regimen. This is probably the single most important factor in treatment, particularly with Grade I and Grade II injuries. Many of the problems resulting from ankle sprains are due to the presence of blood and edema in and around the joint. This restricts the range of motion of the joint and can act as an irritant causing excessive synovial reaction. As well as ice, compression and elevation, it is important for the injured athlete to avoid factors which will promote blood flow and swelling, e.g. hot showers, heat rubs, alcohol, excessive weight bearing.

Reduction of pain and swelling

Pain and swelling can be reduced with the use of electrotherapeutic modalities, e.g., *tens*, interferential, magnetic field therapy. Analgesics may be required. Gentle soft tissue therapy and mobilization after the first 48 hours also may help to reduce pain. By reducing pain and swelling, muscle inhibition around the joint is minimized enabling range of motion exercises to be performed.

Restoration of full range of motion

The patient may be non weight bearing on crutches for the first 24 hours, but should then commence partial weight bearing in normal heel-toe gait. It will be necessary from this stage to protect the damaged joint with strapping or bracing. This will allow partial and ultimately full weight bearing without danger of aggravating the injury. Accessory and physiological mobilization of the ankle, subtalar and midtarsal joints should be commenced early in the rehabilitation process. As soon as pain allows, active range of motion exercises, e.g. stationary cycling, can be commenced.

Muscle conditioning

Strengthening exercises should be commenced as soon as pain allows. Active exercises should be performed initially with gradually increasing resistance. Exercises should include plantar and dorsiflexion, inversion and eversion. Eversion strength is particularly important in the prevention of future lateral ligament injuries. Weight bearing exercises should be commenced as soon as possible.

Restoration of normal proprioception

Proprioception is invariably impaired after ankle ligament

injuries. Proprioceptive retraining exercises can be commenced early in the rehabilitation stage and should be gradually progressed from balancing on one leg to the use of the rockerboard or minitramp and ultimately to functional activities while balancing.

Functional exercises, e.g., jumping, hopping, twisting, figure-of-eight running, should be commenced when the athlete is pain-free, has full range of motion and adequate muscle strength and proprioception.

Return to Sport

Return to sport is permitted when functional exercises can be performed without pain during or after activity. While performing rehabilitation activities and upon return to sport, added ankle protection is required. This can be provided either with taping or bracing. As both seem equally effective, the choice of taping or bracing should be made on the grounds of patient preference, cost, availability and expertise in tape application. Any athlete who has had a significant lateral ligament injury should have protective taping or bracing for all future sporting activities. There are a number of methods to protect against inversion injuries. The three main methods of tape application are stirrups, heel lock and the figure-of-six. Usually at least two of these methods are used. Braces have the advantage of ease of fitting and adjustment, lack of skin irritation and reduced cost compared to taping over a lengthy period. There are a number of different ankle braces available. The lace-up brace is an effective ankle brace.

Treatment of grade III injuries

Treatment of grade III ankle injuries requires initial conservative management over a 6 week period. If the patient continues to make good progress and is able to perform sporting activity with the aid of taping or bracing and without persistent problems during or following activity, surgery may not be required. If however, despite appropriate rehabilitation and protection, the patient complains of recurrent episodes of instability or persistent pain, then surgical reconstruction of the lateral ligament, using one of the peroneal tendons or a fibular periosteal flap, is recommended. Following surgery, it is extremely important to undertake a comprehensive rehabilitation programme to restore full joint range of motion, strength and proprioception. The indications for use of nonsteroidal anti-inflammatory drugs in ankle injuries is unclear. The majority of practitioners tend to prescribe these drugs in all cases of lateral ligament sprains although evidence of their efficacy in this condition is not convincing. However, it may be appropriate to commence medication 2-3 days following injury because of the risk of developing synovitis on resumption of weight bearing.

Medial Ligament Injuries

Medial ligament injuries do not occur as frequently as lateral ligament injuries because the deltoid ligament requires considerable force to be damaged. Occasionally they may be seen in conjunction with a lateral ligament injury. Medial ligament injuries may occur with fracture of the medial malleolus, talar dome or damage to articular surfaces. Medial ligament sprains should be treated in the same manner as lateral ligament sprains, although return to activity may be prolonged.

Pott's fracture

A fracture affecting one or more of the malleoli (lateral, medial, posterior) is known as a Pott's fracture. It can be difficult to distinguish clinically between a fracture and a moderate to severe ligament sprain. Both conditions may result from inversion injuries, with severe pain and varying degrees of swelling and disability. The management of these fractures involves restoration of the normal relationship between the superior surface of the talus and the ankle mortise (inferior margins of tibia and fibula). If this relationship has been disrupted, internal fixation is required. Isolated spiral fractures of the lateral malleolus (without medial ligament instability) and posterior malleolar fractures involving less than 25% of the articular surface are very stable. These fractures can be treated symptomatically with immobilization and crutches in the early stages for pain relief only. Lateral malleolar fractures associated with medial instability, hairline medial malleolar fractures or larger undisplaced posterior malleolar fractures are potentially unstable, but may be treated conservatively. This involves a below knee cast extending to include the metatarsal heads. A walking heel may be applied after swelling has subsided (3-5 days). The cast should be worn for 6 weeks.

Displaced medial malleolar, large posterior malleolar, bimalleolar or trimalleolar fractures, or any displaced fracture which involves the ankle mortise, should be internally fixed. A comprehensive rehabilitation program should be undertaken following surgical fixation or removal of cast. The aims of the rehabilitation program are to restore full range of motion, strengthen the surrounding muscles and improve proprioception.

Persistent pain after Ankle sprain: the "difficult ankle"

In most cases of ligament sprain, the patient progresses satisfactorily through the rehabilitation process with reduction in pain and swelling and improvement in function. However, there is a significant group of patients who do not progress well and complain of persistent pain, swelling and impaired function without any indication of improvement 3-6 weeks after their injury. In these cases, it is important to consider the presence of one of the conditions listed in Table 5.

Table 5: Causes of persistent ankle pain following acute injury

— Inadequate rehabilitation
— Osteochondral fracture of the dome of the talus
— Chronic synovitis of the ankle joint
— Chronic ligamentous instability
— Sinus tarsi syndrome
— Antero-inferior tibiofibular ligament (AITFL) injury
— Anterior impingement syndrome
— Posterior impingement syndrome
— Anterolateral impingement
— Dislocation of the peroneal tendons
— Other fractures
— Avulsion fracture of the base of the 5th metatarsal
— Fracture of the lateral process of the talus
— Fracture of the anterior process of the calcaneus
— Fracture of the tibial plafond
— Fracture of the posterior process of the talus / os Trigonum
— Reflex sympathetic dystrophy (RSD)

An ankle ligament injury which is inadequately rehabilitated may present with persistent pain and loss of function. This usually occurs with increased activity levels. The common problems associated with inadequate rehabilitation are a loss of range of motion in the ankle joint (especially dorsiflexion), weakness of the peroneal muscles and impaired proprioception. Management involves restoration of full dorsiflexion by mobilization of the ankle joint, a programme of strengthening exercises for the peroneal muscles and proprioceptive exercises.If rehabilitation has been appropriate and symptoms persist, it is necessary to consider the presence of other pathology. Symptoms of intra-articular pathology include clicking, locking and joint swelling. Examination may reveal effusion, bony tenderness or swelling at the sinus tarsi or peroneal tendons. The ankle should be re-assessed for evidence of chronic ligamentous instability.

Osteochondral fractures of the talar dome

Osteochondral fractures of the dome of the talus which occur in association with ankle sprains are commonly overlooked. These fractures may occur when there is a compressive component to the inversion injury, especially with landing from a jump. The dome of the talus is compressed by the tibial plafond causing damage of the osteochondral surface. The fractures occur most commonly in the superomedial and the superolateral corners of the talus. If large, these fractures may be recognized at the time of injury. The fracture site will be tender and may be evident on X-ray. Usually the fracture is not detected initially and the patient presents some time later complaining of an unremitting ache in the ankle, despite appropriate treatment for a ankle sprain. The patient often presents with a history of progressing well following a sprain, but then developing symptoms of increasing pain and swelling, stiffness and perhaps catching or locking as activity is increased.

Head Injury

Head injury is one of the most common forms of acquired neurological damage, particularly in young males. Head injuries are especially prevalent in contact sports that produce collisions, in sports where participants move or fall at high velocity and in sports that involve the use of force imparting implements. The incidence is highest in combat sports, such as boxing, where the head is a legitimate target. However, head injury is also common in contact sports such as the various codes of football, especially gridiron, where the annual incidence may be as high as 10 - 20% of participants, and rugby, which has up to twice the risk of other (non gridiron) football codes.

Other non-contact sports with a higher risk of head injury include motor racing, equestrian and gymnastic events, snow, board and blade sports, and cycling. Sports where head injury is rare but potentially severe include golf, shooting, cricket, baseball, and field hockey. The focus in this chapter is on brain injury. However, head injuries often involve significant damage to scalp, skull, meninges and blood vessels as well as the face, jaws, eyes, ears and neck. The most common form of head injury in sport is an episode of concussion, from which a full recovery is usual. However, any head injury can have immediate or delayed life threatening consequences and serious long-term sequelae. As such, all head injuries require thorough systematic assessment by the sports physician:

(a) to recognise and manage the acute consequences, including the prevention of secondary brain damage

(b) to arrange the safe transfer of the injured athlete to an appropriate treatment facility when necessary or

(c) to ensure that the athlete is closely monitored for at least 24 hours and returns to participation only when fully recovered. Finally,

(d) prevention also needs to be addressed by the sports physician. There are five main sections are given below:

— Mechanisms of brain injury, which provides a summary of the anatomical, physiological, and pathological issues that influence management and prevention.

— Clinical features of brain injury, including symptoms and signs of concussion.

— On site assessment and management of head injuries.

— Post acute assessment and management of concussion, which includes clinical and psychometric assessment of recovery and guidelines for the return to participation in sport.

— Prevention measures including athlete preparation, protective devices and rule modifications.

Head injuries in sport usually result from direct impact of the head but can occur when the head is subjected to forces translated from elsewhere on the body. Brain injury may be primary, due to the direct application of physical forces damaging brain and associated vascular tissue, or secondary, arising from intracranial and extracranial complications of injuries to the head and other parts of the body.

Forces producing brain injury

— *Forces acting on the brain produce three types of tissue stress:* compressive, tensile, and shearing. Compressor forces tend to produce focal contusions and if relieved promptly produce the least long-term consequences. Tensile (stretching) forces act mainly on long fibre pathways and damage tends to be more diffuse (diffuse axonal injury). Shearing forces operate parallel to surfaces and can produce serious consequences by tearing brain and vascular tissue.

— Most forces are dynamic and result in propulsion and rotation of the brain within the cranium following impacts to either the head or body. Cerebro spinal fluid (CSF) dissipates focally applied forces and permits gliding of the hemispheres within the cranium.

— A forceful blow to the head usually produces maximal brain injury at the site of impact (coup injury) particularly if the head is stationary before impact. A moving head striking a non-moveable surface, as in falls or collisions, may also produce brain injury at the opposite pole of the cranium (contra coup injury). This is because the brain lags behind in the moving cranium, thereby squeezing protective CSF away from the trailing pole.

— The magnitude of any force is the product of mass and acceleration (Newton's Law). If the neck muscles are tensed at impact, the mass of the head approximates that of the whole body and acceleration (or deceleration) of the head is greatly reduced for any given force. Conversely, when the head is not braced, as in unanticipated blows or further blows in an already stunned state, a given force produces much greater acceleration of the head.

Pathophysiology of primary brain injury

— Gliding of the brain within the cranium is impeded at three main sites (a) dura mater - brain attachments e.g. midline falx cerebri and tentorium cerebelli (b) irregular and protuberant surfaces of the frontal and middle fossa of the base of the skull (c) wherever CSF is dissipated by acceleration, especially at the poles of the frontal and temporal lobes.

— Focal contusions occur mainly at or opposite sites of impact and comprise local petechial haemorrhages and necrotic damage, which are often accompanied by surrounding oedema and subarachnoid haemorrhage.

— Propulsion and rotation of the hemispheres on the relatively fixed brainstem may cause damage to ascending brain stem pathways, ranging from stretching with transient impairment of consciousness to tearing of subcortical fibre tracts with immediate unconsciousness and coma.

— General cerebral oedema due to a combination of local metabolic derangement, breakdown of the blood-brain barrier and obstructions to venous outflow, leads to a rise in intracranial pressure.

Pathophysiology of secondary brain injury

Head injuries may result in complications that are life threatening and can have serious long-term consequences. Because they are often remediable in their early stages, they require immediate attention.

Intracranial complications

Intracranial complications include skull fracture, intracranial haemorrhage, raised intracranial pressure, cerebral hypoxia, and infection.

— Skull fractures may result in direct brain compression, intracranial bleeding, CSF leaks and infection. Brain injury may occur without a skull fracture; however the presence of a skull fracture greatly increases the risk of intracranial bleeding and infection. The site of a fracture is also critical in anticipating complications e.g., temporo-parietal damage to meningeal vessels, frontal damage to sinuses. Fractures may be either of the vault or the base of the skull.

— Vault fractures, which may be linear or depressed, are usually associated with scalp haematomas or a localised area of swelling and tenderness.

— Basal fractures are harder to detect and usually involve intracranial bleeding. Periorbital haematomas, subconjunctival haemorrhage and CSF rhinorrhoea are signs of an anterior fossa fracture; CSF otorrhoea, haemotympanum and retromastoid bruising are signs of a petrous bone fracture.

— Close observation and radiological investigation are required for all suspected skull fractures. Opinions differ on the value of routine CT scan for all mild head injuries. Early CT scan and early discharge of patients with normal radiological and neurological findings has been advocated as being as safe and more cost effective than hospitalization for observation with CT scan performed only after clinical deterioration.

— Intracranial haemorrhage may result in local compression, raised intracranial pressure, and ischaemia to the area of supply of the damaged vessel. All intracranial haematomas constitute a priority in the management of head injury because of their immediate threat to life and eventual recovery of function and because they may be surgically remediable. Haematomas may develop immediately or some time after the initial injury preceded by a lucid interval. Delay in recognising and treating intracranial bleeding is the most common cause of avoidable mortality and morbidity due to head injury. Vigilance needs to be maintained for at least 24 hours. The four types of intracranial haemorrhage are:

a) Extradural haematomas result from shearing forces or skull fractures that tear blood vessels supplying the dura and skull. Haematomas may form rapidly (high pressure bleeding between dura and skull) and compress the brain leading to early loss of consciousness and localising neurological signs or they may occur up to several hours following the initial injury.

b) Subdural haematomas are the most common form of sports related intracranial bleeding. Shearing and direct impact forces tear small veins resulting in low pressure bleeding between the brain and dura matter. Signs and symptoms may be subtle and develop insidiously over days or even weeks.

c) Subarachnoid haemorrhage may result from any head injury, however mild. Severe headache and localising signs usually develop rapidly.

d) Intracerebral haemorrhage occurs with major brain injury. Intraventricular haemorrhage may lead to subsequent blockade of CSF outflow. Brainstem haematomas are life threatening.

— Raised intracranial pressure is a serious consequence of brain injury that may result from several causes including depressed fractures, hypoxia, hypercapnia, hyperperfusion, hypoperfusion, intracranial haemorrhage, and intracranial infection. Raised intracranial pressure leads to cerebral compression, which may be followed by herniation around the brainstem with venous obstruction and infarction. Signs include fluctuations in consciousness, fits and focal neurological deficits.

— Two rare conditions are associated with life threatening rises in intracranial pressure after even minor head injuries.

 — Malignant brain oedema syndrome occurs in children and adolescents as diffuse brain swelling with extreme hyperaemia. It may be due to loss of autoregulation but the mechanism is unknown. After even relatively minor head injury, there is a deterioration of consciousness resembling, in its rapidity, extradural bleeds in adults. Prompt intubation and measures to reduce intracranial pressure such as hyperventilation and osmotic diuretics are required. The mortality rate is high.

  - Second impact syndrome is a variant of malignant brain oedema syndrome that is seen in adults following even minor head trauma when still suffering symptoms of a previous head injury. Loss of autoregulation precipitated by an unknown mechanism leads to massive and diffuse hyperaemia and oedema of the brain. Intracranial pressure rises within minutes and may lead to herniation and coma. Prompt measures to maintain respiration and reduce intracranial pressure as above are indicated. The mortality rate approaches 50% and morbidity is near to 100%.

- Hypoxia due to loss of CNS control of airway patency and breathing may occur following either serious primary injury to the brain stem or may be secondary to raised intracranial pressure with brain herniation. Brain hypoxia may also result from extracranial complications.

- Infection (meningitis or brain abscess) may occur when the dura is penetrated. Direct contamination of the intracranial cavity may occur in compound depressed fractures of the vault, whereas contact with middle ear cavity and nasal sinuses may introduce infection in basal fractures.

- Concussive convulsions seen within seconds of insult are to be distinguished from later epileptic seizures. Such concussive convulsions are rare, transient and do not necessarily lead to the development of epilepsy.

— Post-traumatic epilepsy may develop within days to months. It usually follows traumatic brain injury with prolonged periods of unconsciousness, and occurs in about 23% of hospital admissions of sports-related head injury.

Extracranial complications

Extracranial complications of head or associated injuries may interfere with brain metabolism and perfusion. Given the immediate dependency of brain tissue on its oxygen supply and the potential for remediation of many of the complications, recognition and management of extracranial causes of secondary brain damage constitutes a clinical priority. Causes include injuries interfering with ventilation, such as chest, neck or facial injuries that obstruct airways and affect chest movement, and injuries interfering with brain circulation by producing haemodynamic instability and hypovolaemia.

Non-traumatic sports related brain injury

There are two main causes of non-traumatic sports related brain injury. Cerebral air embolism unique to underwater diving, second most common cause of death after drowning :

— occurs in rapid ascents from > 10 metres

— symptoms may occur within moments to hours of surfacing

— signs include: seizure, hemiplegia, diplopia, tunnel vision, vertigo, or dysarthria

— if diver surfaces unconscious, diagnosis is strong presumption

— seek to recompress subject as soon as possible

High-altitude cerebral oedema accounts for up to 5% of deaths above 4000 metres

— symptoms develop within 72 hours and include ataxia, vertigo, confusion, and hallucinations

— immediate treatment is return to lower elevation and oxygenate

— monitor for signs of raised intracranial pressure and treat accordingly.

Eye Injury

Although the eye accounts for only 0.002% of the body's surface area and has many protective mechanisms including rapid reflex lid closure, production of tears, and protection by bony orbital ridges, eye injuries due to sport are nevertheless common, accounting for one to two per cent of all sports injuries. High risk sports include basketball, squash, and contact sports such as football and boxing. A thorough examination is required for all eye injuries, even those that appear to be minor. All serious eye injuries and ideally all eye injuries should be examined by an ophthalmologist, but this is not always possible or practical. The clinician dealing with eye injuries must therefore have a thorough knowledge of the anatomy and physiology of the eye, and be able to treat minor eye injuries whilst being able to recognize and refer serious injuries to an ophthalmologist.

Necessary equipment

— ophthalmoscope, torch, visual acuity card, and eyelid speculum
— sterile single use vials of fluorescein stain, mydriatic drops, anaesthetic drops and saline for irrigation
— sterile eye pads, eye shield (plastic/metal), cotton-tipped swabs, and tape

In all eye injuries a thorough history detailing the mechanism of injury is vital. Of most importance is visual status - whether there has been any decrease in visual acuity after the injury. It is also important to ask what the patient's visual acuity prior to the injury was like. A detailed history should include:

— *Symptoms experienced:* Ask the patient whether there is pain, blurred vision, double vision, or a decrease in visual acuity. Photophobia is suggestive of traumatic iritis whilst floaters and flashing lights suggest a retinal detachment, tear, or vitreous haemorrhage. Diplopia is associated with blowout fractures. Loss of consciousness or altered mental status suggests significant trauma and additional injuries. Ask whether there has been any discharge, tearing, itching, burning, redness, headache, or altered facial sensation.

— *Mechanism of injury*—velocity of injury causing particles, nature of particles involved, blunt injury versus projectiles, whether protective equipment was worn at time of injury.

— *Ophthalmic history*—previous eye injuries and eye problems, and whether spectacles or contact lenses are worn normally.

Eye Examination

In order to perform a satisfactory eye examination a clean location with good illumination is required. A thorough eye examination should always be performed with the unaffected eye used for comparison. The following routine is suggested:

— Visual acuity should be tested first as other examinations may require the instillation of mydriatics. The exception to this rule is chemical injuries where irrigation of the eye takes precedence over examination. Visual acuity is tested using a Snellen chart or card. If unavailable a newspaper should be used. Each eye should be tested individually, while the other is covered by a small card or the palm of the hand, using the best corrected vision. A patient unable to read the largest letter should be asked to count the number of fingers the examiner holds up. If this cannot be done then the perception of hand movement should be tested. Failing this perception of light using a torch should be tested.

— Inspect the eyelids for lacerations, haemotoma and bruising.

— Evert the eyelids (instruct the patient to look down with their chin elevated) and inspect the conjuctival sac for signs of trauma and for foreign bodies.

— Examine the cornea and sclera for surface irregularities, perforations, subconjuctival haemorrhages, iris prolapses, and foreign bodies. A magnifying lens or ophthalmoscope should be used. Fluorescein dye may aid in outlining corneal abrasions, which appear bright green under blue cobalt light.

— Examine the anterior chamber. Any haziness, the presence of blood and the depth should be noted. Examine the optic disc and retina. Look for the red reflex (reduced with retinal detachment, haemorrhage, or cataract). A thorough ocular examination should also include examination with a slit lamp.

— Inspect pupils. Note size and shape. Test light reflexes - direct and consensual responses, and perform the swinging torch test.

— Compare the iris colours of each eye and look for iridodonesis (trembling of the iris with quick visual movements due to lack of support e.g. in lens subluxation).

— Examine visual fields carefully and note any defects.

— Examine the face looking for signs of orbital fractures, nerve palsies, and altered face sensation.

— General examination. Ensure that no other more urgent injuries have been sustained.

The Face

Maxillofacial injuries in sport are usually the result of direct trauma and include fractures of the facial skeleton, intra- and extraoral lacerations, and dental trauma. Although face masks, helmets and mouth guards have reduced the number of facial injuries in sports such as American football, cricket, and ice hockey1, the incidence of facial injuries is still significant.

Fractures of the mandible

Fractures of the mandible are the most common maxillofacial injury from sport and are usually the result of a direct blow. Mandibular fracture patterns include condyle, angle, body, symphysis, ramus (rare) and coronoid process (rare).

Condylar fractures

The condyle is the most common site of mandibular fracture. Most fractures are sub-condylar fracturing through the weak area at the neck of the condyle. The fracture may be undisplaced, displaced (anterior-medially due to pull of the lateral pterygoid muscle, condyle remains within the glenoid fossa), or dislocated. Symptoms - pain and tenderness from the tempero-mandibular joint, exacerbated if the patient opens his mouth or clenches his teeth. Signs - swelling in front of the ear, alteration of the natural bite (occluded) position with gagging of the posterior molars, deviation in mandibular movements on opening towards the side of the fracture. Investigations - the diagnosis is frequently missed.

The orthopantomogram (OPG) and posterior-anterior (PA) mandible x-ray must be carefully studied by outlining the contour of the condyles bilaterally. Treatment - maintenance of the airway is the first priority in fractures of the mandible. If the patient is conscious they should be advised to support the lower jaw with their hands in a forward sitting position. If the fracture is comminuted or displaced then a bandage or cervical collar may be applied taking care not to compromise the airway by causing backward displacement of the mandible. Unconscious patients should be placed in a lateral ('coma') position so that blood and saliva can drain from the mouth. The mouth should be cleared of any dislodged teeth, dentures, blood and other foreign bodies then the head tilted and jaw supported.

In children management of condylar fractures is non-surgical because remodeling occurs with complete regeneration of the normal condylar anatomy. Jaw exercises to achieve normal occlusion is usually all that is required. If normal occlusion is not consistently attainable then intermaxillary fixation for 2 weeks followed by a period of guiding elastics may be required.

In adults, the management of sub-condylar fracture is controversial. There are opposing views on whether displaced condylar fractures should be treated by open or closed reduction. Lim suggests that open reduction should be reserved for gross fracture dislocations and when correct occlusion can not be attained by closed reduction.

In the majority of cases of condylar fracture in adults there is minimal alteration to the occlusion position. The patient is able to achieve a correct occlusion with a minimum of effort and simple jaw exercises may be all that is required to achieve a consistent occlusion. Good results have been achieved by both conservative management and open reduction but it seems preferable to avoid surgery if it is possible to do so without compromise to the outcome. If the occlusion is not readily achieved then this is an indication for closed reduction. Arched bars are placed and the patient is placed into intermaxillary fixation for a period of two weeks after which it is released and guiding elastics used for a further two to four weeks.

Fractures of the angle

The angle is the second most common site of mandibular fracture, usually occurring through the unerupted lower third molar. A concomitant body fracture or sub-condylar fracture contralaterally may be present. Bilateral angle fractures are not common.

*Symptoms:*the patient will state that their bit feels different from normal (change in occlusion). There may also be altered sensation of the lower lip and chin due to injury to the inferior alveolar nerve.

Signs—the teeth do not interdigitate well into the occlusion.

Fractures of the body

Fracture of the body of the mandible may be midline (symphyseal), lateral to the midline (parasymphyseal), or midbody (molar and premolar area). Symphyseal fractures usually present with little displacement. They are difficult to demonstrate an X-ray.

Parasymphyseal fractures usually present with considerable displacement and can be very mobile.

Clinical features—there is pain and discomfort as well as swelling and ecchymosis. There may be loose teeth present on either side of the fracture.

Treatment—with undisplaced surgery is not usually required. Treatment is with antibiotics, a soft diet and regular review. The treatment for displaced fracture is open reduction and fixation. Whılst the patient is awaiting definitive surgery, stabilization of the fracture with a simple wire passed interdentally and on either side of the fracture can improve patient comfort. Post-operative care includes antibiotics, a soft diet, strict oral hygiene and avoidance of contact sports for at least 6 weeks.

Midbody fractures are usually unilateral and present with very little displacement since the muscles on either side of the fracture site have a counteracting action on each other.

8

Exercise Science in Sports

Aging and Exercise

Aging and ultimate death seem characteristic of all living organisms. Atherosclerosis and arteriosclerosis progressively decrease the tissue oxygen supply, and in some organs such as the brain, cells that die are not replaced. In other tissues, the cell constituents change with aging; for example, cross-linkages develop between adjacent collagen fibrils, decreasing their elasticity and facilitating mechanical injury. In consequence, most biological functions show a progressive, age-related deterioration. The mechanisms underlying the aging process are not well understood. Possible hypotheses include a "wear and tear" which exceeds the reparative capacity of the tissues, a development of immunity to the individual's own protein constituents, and errors in cell division, associated with exposure to external radiation or endogenous mitogens such as peroxidases. Some biologists have even argued that aging has been "programmed" by evolution to avoid the hazard of overpopulation.

Age Classification

Young adulthood typically covers the period from 20-35 years of age, when both biological function and physical performance reach their peak. During young middle-age (35-45 years), physical activity usually wanes, with a 5-10 kg accumulation of body fat. Active pursuits may be shared with a growing family, but it becomes less important to impress either an employer or persons of the opposite sex with physical appearance and performance. During later middle-age (45-65 years), women reach the menopause, and men also substantially reduce their output of sex hormones. Career opportunities have commonly peaked, and a larger disposable income often allows energy demanding domestic tasks to be deputed to service contractors. The decline in physical condition thus continues and may accelerate.

In early old age (65-75 years), there may be a modest increase of physical activity, in an attempt to fill free time resulting from retirement (8). By middle old age (75-85 years), many people have developed some physical disability, and in the final stage (very old age, over 85 years) they become totally dependent. A typical expectation is of 8-10 years of partial disability, and a year of total dependency. There are nevertheless wide inter-individual differences in functional status at any given chronological age. In terms of maximal oxygen intake, muscle strength and flexibility, the best preserved 65-year-old may out-perform a sedentary 25-year-old. Whether assessing fitness for continuing employment or recommending an exercise prescription, decisions should thus be based upon biological rather than chronological age.

Unfortunately, there is no very satisfactory method of determining a person's biological age, because the different biological systems age at differing rates. Attempts to combine such measurements as graying of the hair, loss of skin elasticity, a decrease of vital capacity, and a decrease of reaction time into a global index seem to provide no more than a complicated and inaccurate method of assessing the individual's chronological age.

Aging and Energy Consumption

A major fraction of total daily energy demand arises from resting metabolism, and it is thus important to note that resting metabolism decreases with aging, by about 10% from early adulthood to the age of retirement, and a further 10% subsequently. One reason is the loss of metabolically active muscle mass and parallel increase in metabolically inert depot fat. In later old age, there may also be some overall reduction in cellular metabolism. Food intake must be correspondingly adjusted if body fat is not to increase further. A low total intake of food may fail to satisfy daily requirements of protein and other key nutrients, particularly calcium. One important by-product of a physical activity program for the older senior is thus an increased intake of key nutrients without recourse to the provision of synthetic dietary supplements.

Aging and Aerobic Performance

The maximal oxygen intake declines by about 5 $ml.kg^{-1}.min^{-1}$ per decade from 25 to 65 years of age, with some possible acceleration thereafter. It is difficult to be certain how much of this loss is inevitable, and the extent to which the decline results from a progressive decrease of habitual physical activity; ordinary people certainly become more sedentary as they age and even older athletes usually reduce the rigor of their training. There have been occasional claims that individuals who become vigorously physically active can sustain an unchanged maximal oxygen intake for many years, but a critical review of the data suggests that once such subjects have realized any immediate training response, they resume a relatively normal rate of aging. Even in athletes who maintain their daily training volume, the rate of decrease of maximal oxygen intake is only a little slower than in the general population. Potential causes of the age-related loss in aerobic power include decreases in maximal heart rate, stroke volume and arterio-venous oxygen difference.

Heart Rate

Maximal heart rate decreases mainly because of a decreased responsiveness to circulating catecholamines. The classical equation [peak rate = (220 - age in years)] implies a maximum of about 155 beats.min^{-1} at age 65 years. More recent research suggests that a well-motivated 65-year-old can attain a rate of 170 beats. min^{-1} or more during uphill treadmill running, although muscle weakness may lead to somewhat lower maxima during cycle ergometry. Peak values are further reduced if the subject experiences breathlessness (in chronic pulmonary disease) or develops myocardial ischemia (in the sick sinus syndrome).

Some argued that if care was taken to exclude subjects with myocardial ischemia, the heart of a typical 65-year-old subject could compensate for a low maximal beating rate by increasing the end-diastolic volume and thus cardiac stroke volume. However, their view has not been confirmed by subsequent research. During submaximal exercise, the stroke volume may be greater than in a younger adult, but an elderly person has difficulty in sustaining stroke volume as maximal effort is approached. There are many constraints upon peak ventricular function in the elderly. Venous filling is impaired by poor peripheral venous tone, varicosities, and a slow relaxation of the ventricular wall. Reduced sensitivity to catecholamines blunts the inotropic increase of myocardial contractility during vigorous exercise. After-loading of the ventricle also rises more than in a younger individual, in part because of hypertension and a loss of arterial elasticity, and in part because weakened skeletal muscles must contract at a larger fraction of their peak voluntary force. Finally, ventricular contractility may be impaired by the development of silent myocardial ischemia.

The maximal arterio-venous oxygen difference decreases from perhaps 140-150 $ml.dL^{-1}$ in a young adult to 120-130 $ml.dL^{-1}$ in a senior citizen. This change reflects the direction of a larger fraction of the total cardiac output of the exerciser to regions (the skin and the viscera) where oxygen extraction is quite limited.

Depending on the nature of the task and the working environment, sustained exercise is fatiguing if it demands more than 33-50% of the person's maximal oxygen intake. Thus, the aging of oxygen transport progressively restricts the ability of the senior citizen to undertake the normal activities of daily living such as walking up a slight rise. Full independence probably requires a peak oxygen transport of 12-14 ml/[kg.min]. The maximal oxygen intake of many seniors drops below this threshold around 80 years of age, the final precipitant of dependence being the added loss of function caused by a period of bed rest for some inter-current illness.

Age and Training Response

An appropriately graded aerobic training program can augment the aerobic power of 65 year old subjects by as much as 10 $ml.kg^{-1}.min^{-1}$ over a 3 month period, effectively reducing the biological age of the oxygen transporting system by 20 years. A lack of aerobic power thus should not limit the independence of a well-trained, active individual unless she or he survives to the unlikely age of 100 years. Aerobic training eliminates premature disability, but has little influence on survival beyond the age of 80 years. Rather, it induces a "squaring" of morbidity and mortality curves, so that good health is preserved until shortly before death. Activity patterns in late middle age are quite strong predictors of the likelihood of dependency as a senior. Because initial fitness is quite low, the aerobic condition of a senior can be improved by low intensity of training. Gains are greatest if a heart rate of 130-140 $beats.min^{-1}$ can be sustained, but useful if slower progress is seen with regular training at heart rates of 110-120 $beats.min^{-1}$. In the frail elderly, heart rates rarely exceed 85 $beats.min^{-1}$, and some training response may then be anticipated even with activities inducing a heart rate of only 100 $beats.min^{-1}$.

Aging and Musculo-Skeletal Function

Muscles

Strength peaks around 25 years of age, plateaus through

35 or 40 years of age, and then shows an accelerating decline, with 25% loss of peak force by the age of 65 years. Muscle mass decreases, apparently with a selective loss in the cross-section if not the numbers of type II fibers. It is unclear whether there is a general hypotrophy of skeletal muscle, or a selective hypoplasia and degeneration of Type II fibers, associated with a loss of nerve terminal sprouting. Other possible causes of functional loss include a deterioration of end-plate structures, impaired excitation-contraction coupling, and decreased fiber recruitment. Both contraction time and half-relaxation time are prolonged, and maximal contraction velocity is decreased. Changes are greater in the legs than in the arms, possibly because there is a greater decrease in use of the legs with aging. Muscular endurance at a given fraction of maximal voluntary force apparently improves with age, in part because the muscles now contain a larger proportion of type I fibers and in part because weaker muscle contractions restrict perfusion less than in a younger person. Loss of strength progressively impedes every day living. It becomes difficult to carry a 5 kg bag of groceries, to open a vial of medicine, and even to lift the body mass from a toilet seat. The male/female strength ratio is unchanged, so that women are limited by a loss of strength at an earlier age than men.

Muscle strength can be greatly improved by as little as 8 weeks of resisted training, even in 90 year old subjects. Protein synthesis proceeds more slowly than in a younger adult, but cross-sectional comparisons between active and inactive individuals suggest that much of the wasting of lean tissue can be avoided by regular resisted exercise. Stronger muscles further enhance function by stabilizing osteo-arthritic joints, reducing the risk of falls, and lessening the extent of dyspnea. At one time, it was feared that resisted exercise might cause a dangerous rise of blood pressure, provoking a heart attack. However, if the subject avoids performing a Valsalva maneuver and individual contractions are held for no more than a few seconds at 60% of peak voluntary force, the rise of blood pressure is no greater than would be anticipated during a typical bout of cycle ergometer exercise.

Flexibility

The elasticity of tendons, ligaments and joint capsules is decreased as cross-linkages develop between adjacent fibrils of collagen. Over the span of working life, adults lose some 8-10 cm of lower-back and hip flexibility, as measured by the "sit-and- reach" test. The restriction in the range of movement at the major joints becomes yet more pronounced during retirement, and eventually, independence is threatened because the subject cannot climb into a car or a normal bath, ascend a small step, or complete the movements required for dressing and combing the hair. Flexibility is thought to be conserved or improved by gently taking the main joints through their full range of motion each day. If muscle weakness and arthritis are already advanced, such activities are best attempted in warm water. Buoyancy then supports body-weight, and warmth increases the immediate flexibility of the joints.

Bone Structure

There is a progressive decrease in the calcium content and a deterioration in the organic matrix of the bones with aging. However, the dividing line between normality and pathology is unclear, and it is also uncertain how far a decrease of habitual physical activity contributes to the age-related calcium loss. Changes are more marked in women than in men, due in part to sex differences in the hormone profile and in part to a lower intake of calcium and good quality protein in women. The calcium loss can begin as early as 30 years, and in women the process accelerates for some 5 years around the menopause. In later old age, the bones become so weak that a mild fall, a bout of coughing, or even a vigorous muscle contraction can cause a "pathological" fracture. A fracture of the hip quite commonly initiates irreversible bed rest and death. A deterioration of the vertebrae also contributes to senile kyphosis.

Regular load-bearing exercise can halt and sometimes even reverse bone mineral loss through the eighth decade of life. Such a regimen is particularly effective when accompanied by a high calcium diet (1500 mg/day). In women, many authorities also recommend the administration of estrogens, although the risks of such therapy require further assessment.

Aging and Metabolic Function

Many hormonal control mechanisms work less efficiently in an older person. For example, the pancreas and the thyroid are affected by damage to and/or a decrease in the number of secreting cells, and the ventricular muscle has a decrease in the number or the affinity of catecholamine receptors. Clinical consequences of these hormonal changes include the development of maturity-onset diabetes, and myxedema, with resulting obesity, poor cold tolerance and depression. Diabetes mellitus presents immediate risks of ketosis, hyperglycemia and hypoglycemia. Long-term complications (skin infections, ulcers, peripheral vascular arteriosclerosis, myocardial ischemia, peripheral neuropathy, retinopathies and cataract formation) can also limit the subject's exercise tolerance. However, moderate exercise with some restriction of energy intake is an effective treatment for maturity-onset diabetes mellitus; many patients are thus spared the complication of long-term insulin therapy and rigid control of food intake. Exercise may also correct both obesity and depression in the patient with hypothyroidism.

Athletic Performance

The age of peak athletic performance depends upon the key functional element required of the successful competitor. In events where flexibility is paramount (for example, gymnastics and brief swimming events) the top competitors are commonly adolescents. In aerobic events, performance usually peaks in the mid-twenties, as gains from prolonged training, improved mechanical skills and competitive experience are negated by decreases in maximal oxygen intake and flexibility. Because of a longer plateauing of muscle strength, performance in anaerobic events declines less steeply, and in pursuits such as golf and equitation, where experience is paramount, the best competitors are aged 30-40 years. Caution is needed in drawing physiological inferences from athletic records, since the pool of potential competitors decreases with age. Moreover, the motives of older participants often change from competitive success (winning at all costs) to social interaction, and some participants in Masters events lack cumulated skills, since they did not begin competing until they reached their late thirties.

Risks of Exercise

The risk of a cardiac emergency is increased substantially when a person is actually exercising. Some physicians have thus argued that older people who intend to exercise should undergo exhaustive preliminary screening, including an exercise electrocardiogram. This may be desirable if the person intends to embark on very strenuous competitive training, but it is undesirable if an older individual merely wishes to make a small increase in their habitual daily physical activity.

It is usually difficult to motivate older people to exercise regularly. Insistence on extensive screening suggests that physical activity is dangerous, and creates additional barriers of cost and time which reduce the likelihood that an intention to exercise will result in active exercise behavior. In fact, the interpretation of exercise ECGs is very difficult in many elderly persons, and there is little evidence that either a clinical evaluation or a stress electrocardiogram can detect those who will have an adverse exercise outcome. Moreover, the person who begins an exercise program is at a lower overall risk of sudden death than a sedentary peer, and perhaps because of a less ambitious attitude toward exercise, the relative risks of physical activity (deaths when exercising vs deaths when sedentary) decrease rather than increase as a person becomes older. Finally, if a well-loved form of exercise does provoke sudden death in an 80-year-old, this is a more pleasant end than many alternative ways of dying. Nevertheless, certain precautions can increase the safety of exercise for the older individual.

The recommended dose of exercise should do no more than leave the participant pleasantly tired on the following day. Recovery processes proceed slowly, and vigorous training should thus be pursued on alternate days. In individuals with pre-existing articular disease, walking should be substituted for jogging or running; fast walking offers an adequate training stimulus, with less risk of slipping, and a much smaller impact stress on the knees. Weight-supported activities such as swimming and aquabics are particularly helpful for those with joint problems. Vision, hearing and balance are all poorer than in a younger person.

The senior should thus avoid sports where there is a risk of collision with opponents or stationary objects. If there is a history of falls, special care is needed in pursuing activities that require a good sense of balance (whether climbing, skiing and cycling, or merely walking on a slippery pool deck). In older people taking hypotensive medication, there is a danger of a sudden loss of consciousness when standing at the end of a bout of exercise, particularly if the room is hot, or the veins are relaxed by a period in a pool. Environmental extremes are poorly tolerated, and if the weather is extremely hot or cold, activity should be taken inside an air-conditioned facility (for example, rapid walking in an indoor shopping mall). For those who are extremely frail, some physical conditioning can be achieved using exercises taken from a sitting position.

Exercise training cannot restore tissue that has already been destroyed, but it can protect the individual against a number of the chronic diseases of old age. More importantly, it maximizes residual function. In some instances, biological age is reduced by as much as 20 years. Life expectancy is increased, partial and total disability are delayed, and there are major gains in quality-adjusted life expectancy. Exercise is thus a very important component of healthy living for the senior citizen.

Adipose tissue

Adipose tissue is specialized connective tissue that functions as the major storage site for fat in the form of triglycerides. Adipose tissue is found in mammals in two different forms: white adipose tissue and brown adipose tissue. The presence, amount, and distribution of each varies depending upon the species. White adipose tissue serves three functions: heat insulation, mechanical cushion, and most importantly, a source of energy. Subcutaneous adipose tissue, found directly below the skin, is an especially important heat insulator in the body, because it conducts heat only one third as readily as other tissues. The degree of insulation is dependent upon the thickness of this fat layer. For example, a person with a 2-mm layer of subcutaneous fat will feel as comfortable at 15°C as a person with a 1-mm layer at 16°C. Adipose tissue also surrounds internal organs and provides some protection for these organs from jarring.

As the major form of energy storage, fat provides a buffer for energy imbalances when energy intake is not equal to energy output. It is an efficient way to store excess energy, because it is stored with very little water. Consequently, more energy can be derived per gram of fat (9 $kcal.gm^{-1}$) than per gram of carbohydrate (4 $kcal.gm^{-1}$) or protein (4 $kcal.gm^{-1}$). In addition, if terrestrial animals stored their excess energy as carbohydrate, the increased mass would interfere with mobility. The average woman with 20% body fat has about one month of energy stored as fat. There are some constraints on the use of fat as fuel.

Most animals cannot convert lipid into carbohydrate. Tissues that function predominantly anaerobically (e.g.. erythrocytes) must rely on carbohydrate for energy and need to have an ample supply available. Additionally, under normal conditions the brain is dependent upon glucose for energy and does not use fatty acids. In unusual metabolic circumstances, the brain can use ketone bodies (a by-product of incomplete fat metabolism) when they are present in sufficiently high quantities. Finally, a typical diet contains a high proportion of carbohydrate, and the transport of insoluble lipids through blood requires a specific mechanism, so it may be "easier" metabolically for tissues to use glucose under typical dietary conditions. Brown adipose tissue, which derives its color from rich vascularization and densely packed mitochondria, is found in various locations, depending upon the species and/or age of the animal. In the rat, brown adipose tissue is found primarily in the interscapular region and the axillae, minor amounts are found near the thymus and in the dorsal midline region of the thorax and abdomen.

During maturation, in non-hibernating animals, brown adipose tissue is metabolically less active, although cold exposure can activate it. In hibernating animals and neonates, brown adipose tissue is important for regulating body temperature via non-shivering thermogenesis. Instead of serving as a substrate, the lipid in brown adipose tissue releases energy directly as heat and is, therefore used in heat production for non-shivering thermogenesis and for utilization of excess caloric intake via diet-induced-thermogenesis. The mechanism of heat generation is related to the metabolism of the mitochondria. Mitochondria from brown adipose tissue have a specific carrier called uncoupling protein that transfers protons from outside to inside without subsequent production of ATP.

Morphology and Development of Adipose Tissue

In adult mammals, the major bulk of adipose tissue is a loose association of lipid-filled cells called adipocytes, which are held in a framework of collagen fibers. In addition to adipocytes, adipose tissue contains stromal-vascular cells including fibroblastic connective tissue cells, leukocytes, macrophages, and pre-adipocytes (not yet filled with lipid), which contribute to structural integrity.

Approximately 60 to 85% of the weight of white adipose tissue is lipid, with 90-99% being triglyceride. Small amounts of free fatty acids, diglyceride, cholesterol, phospholipid and minute quantities of cholesterol ester and monoglyceride are also present. In this lipid mixture, six fatty acids make up approximately 90% of the total, and these are myristic, plamitic, palmitoleic, stearic, oleic, and linoleic. Varying the composition of your diet can vary the fatty acid profile in adipose tissue. The remaining weight of white adipose tissue is composed of water (5 to 30%) and protein (2 to 3%). White adipose tissue is not as richly vascularized as brown adipose tissue, but each adipocyte in white adipose tissue is in contact with at least one capillary. This blood supply provides sufficient support for the active metabolism, which occurs in the thin rim of cytoplasm surrounding the lipid droplet. Blood flow to adipose tissue varies depending upon body weight and nutritional state, with blood flow increasing during fasting. Adipocytes are considered to originate from fibroblast-like precursor cells that differentiate into adipocytes under the appropriate stimulatory conditions.

The precursor cells do not possess any morphological or enzymatic marker that can be used to determine whether they will become adipocytes. The criteria used to identify adipocytes depends upon lipid accumulation within the cell after proliferation has stopped, making early identification of adipocytes difficult. The size of adipose tissue mass is a function of both adipocyte number and size. An increase in adipose tissue mass can occur by hyperplastic growth, which is an increase in the number of adipocytes. This increase in number occurs primarily by mitotic activity in precursor cells.

Adipose tissue mass can also increase by hypertrophic growth, which is an increase in the size of adipocytes. This increase in size occurs primarily by lipid accumulation within the cell. Growth of this tissue in the rat occurs in well-defined stages. From birth to 4 weeks of age, adipose tissue growth is hyperplastic. Overfeeding a rat during this period can lead to permanent increases in body weight and fat cell number. From 4 to 14 weeks of age both adipocyte hypertrophy and hyperplasia occur. Following 14 weeks of age, adipose tissue growth occurs predominantly by adipocyte hypertrophy. The developmental sequence of adipose tissue in humans is less well defined. In contrast to most neonates, the human neonate is born relatively fat. Two periods of hyperplastic growth are probably during the third trimester of pregnancy and just prior to and during puberty.

Contrary to earlier belief, hyperplastic growth can also occur in adulthood (in both humans and rats). When adipocytes fill with lipid and get to a critical size, precursor cells are stimulated to differentiate, and an increase in adipocyte number results. This critical size probably does not occur with moderate overfeeding unless the overfeeding is of long duration. In addition, there are probably individual differences in the size that will result in new adipocyte formation. Once new adipocytes are formed, they remain throughout life and only a reduction in size of the cell is possible. This increased number of adipocytes has far-reaching consequences for the treatment and prevention of obesity.

Adipose-Tissue Metabolism

Lipogenesis

Lipogenesis is the deposition of fat. This process occurs in adipose tissue and in the liver at cytoplasmic and mitochondrial sites

Energy ingested as fat beyond that needed for current energy demands is stored in adipose tissue. In addition, carbohydrate and protein consumed in the diet can be converted to fat. Energy ingested as carbohydrate can be stored as glycogen in the liver and muscle. Carbohydrate can also be converted to triglycerides primarily in the liver and transferred to adipose tissue for storage. Amino acids from ingested proteins are used for new protein synthesis or they can be converted to carbohydrate and fat. Fatty acids, in the form of triglycerides or free fatty acids bound to albumin, are ingested in the diet or synthesized by the liver. Very little synthesis of free fatty acids occurs in the adipocytes. Triglycerides are the most significant source of fatty acids, because this is the form in which dietary lipids are assembled by the gut and liver. Triglycerides made up of long chain fatty acids, in the form of chylomicrons (from intestinal absorption) or lipoproteins (from hepatic synthesis), are hydrolyzed to glycerol and free fatty acids by an enzyme called lipoprotein lipase (LPL). Lipoprotein lipase is synthesized in adipocytes and secreted into adjacent endothelial cells. Chylomicrons and lipoproteins (very low density lipoproteins) contain C-ll apoprotein, which activates LPL. Free fatty acids are taken up by adipocytes in a concentration-dependent manner by a transmembrane transport protein.

Once inside the adipocyte, fatty acids enter a common pool made up of both incoming and outgoing fatty acids. Fatty acids that are stored in the adipose tissue must first combine with coenzyme A to form a thioester and then they are re-esterified in a stepwise manner to triglycerides. Glucose is the primary source of glycerol for this re-esterification process. Only a small amount of glycerol released, when triglycerides are hydrolyzed by LPL, can be reused by adipocytes to form alpha glycerol phosphate to be used for trigyceride assembly. Most glycerol is returned to the circulation. Insulin, a hormone secreted by the beta cells of the pancreas, plays a predominant role in the lipogenic process. The net effect of insulin is to enhance storage and block mobilization and oxidation of fatty acids. Insulin exerts its effect by stimulating LPL formation, so that circulating triglycerides are hydrolyzed and free fatty acids can enter the adipocyte. Insulin is also required for the transport of glucose, which is needed for re-esterification of the triglycerides once inside the adipocyte. Finally, the conversion of glucose to fatty acids is accomplished by insulin's activation of several enzymes.

Lipolysis

Lipolysis is the chemical decomposition and release of fat from adipose tissue. This process predominates over lipogenesis when additional energy is required. The triglycerides within the adipocyte are acted upon by a multi-enzyme complex called hormone sensitive lipase

(HSL), which hydrolyzes the triglyceride into free fatty acids and glycerol. These lipases act consecutively on triglycerides, diglycerides, and monoglycerides. Triglyceride lipase regulates the rate of lipolysis, because its activity is low. Once triglycerides are hydrolyzed to fatty acids and glycerol, fatty acids enter the common free fatty acid pool where they may be re-esterified, undergo beta-oxidation (metabolic degradation), or be released into the circulation as substrates for skeletal muscle, cardiac muscle, and liver. If the fatty acids are to undergo beta-oxidation for ATP production, fatty acids move from the adipocytes into the blood and are carried to the tissues that can use them as an energy source. Long-chain fatty acids enter the cells of these tissues by passive diffusion, and their rate of uptake is proportional to their difference in concentration inside and outside of the cell. Once inside the cells, beta-oxidation begins with "activation", that is, the formation of thioesters with coenzyme A. This activation step converts the fatty acids to a form that is more amenable to the successive biochemical changes that ultimately result in ATP formation.

Insulin reduces mobilization of fatty acids from adipose tissue by inhibiting triglyceride lipase. The mechanism of this inhibition may be through a decrease in cyclic AMP which in turn results in an inhibition of cyclic-AMP-dependent protein kinase. This suppression of lipolysis lowers the rate of fatty acid delivery to the liver and to peripheral tissues. The consequence of fewer fatty acids to the liver is a reduction in the formation of ketoacids (e.g., ketones). Insulin also stimulates the use of ketoacids by peripheral tissues, preventing an accumulation of these acids in the blood.

Adipose Tissue Distribution

Even the most casual observer will note that everyone does not carry their adipose tissue in the same anatomical locations. Adipose tissue that is located predominantly on the upper body has been termed android, male, central, upper-body segment, or "apple" distribution. This distribution pattern is found more frequently in men; consequently the terms android and male. When adipose tissue accumulates predominantly in the lower body, the terms gynoid, female, lower-body segment , or "pear" distribution are used. As the terms gynoid and female imply, this fat pattern is found more frequently in women than in men. What factors determine fat distribution?

A primary factor is genetic background, which can often be seen by looking at the similarity in fat distribution within same-sex family members. As mentioned earlier, gender is also known to affect body fat location. Women usually show greater lower body fat distribution and men show more upper body fat distribution. As an individual ages body fat distribution may change. For example, after the menopause a change towards upper body fat distribution is observed. This change may be due to a relative decrease in LPL activity in the lower body region. Finally, extreme weight gain and weight cycling ("yo-yo dieting") may increase upper body fat.

Upper body fat distribution is correlated with the development of various health problems, including cardiovascular disease, hypertension, and non-insulin dependent diabetes. Excess visceral fat rather than excess upper body subcutaneous fat is associated with increased risk. A quick test to see if you are at risk for complications associated with upper body fat distribution is to calculate your waist-to-hip-ratio by measuring the circumference of your waist and dividing it by the circumference of your hips. Women are at risk if the ratio exceeds 0.85; for men the ratio is 0.95.

Causes of Obesity

Obesity is not a single disorder. A variety of methods and criteria are used to diagnose the presence of obesity. It is the quantity of adipose tissue and not just total body weight that defines obesity. Several factors contribute to the development of obesity: genetics, environment, physiology, psychology, and undetermined. Work from experimental animals shows clear genetic anomalies as one basic cause of obesity. Genes for obesity can be recessive, dominant, or polygenic. Recessive alleles that influence the development of obesity have been identified in various rodents.

In the human population, obesity is a feature of several recessive syndromes, including Bardet-Biedl, Lawrence-Moon, and Prader-Labhart-Willi, as well as, triglyceride storage diseases. These syndromes are relatively rare. A single genetic anomaly in the absence of other concurrent genetic syndromes has yet to be identified in humans. It is possible that alleles at particular loci exert a small effect that is not easily detectable by themselves. If these alleles exist at a large number of loci, collectively they may exert a substantial impact on obesity. Genes clearly influence body size and body fat distribution, and are likely to be involved in modulating human obesity. In humans, it is difficult to separate genetic and environmental factors and assign the relative contribution of each to the development of obesity.

Several familial, twin, and adoption studies have provided a means to study the contributions of heredity and environment. These studies provide strong suggestive data for a genetic component to obesity, as well as modulation of genes by environmental factors. Environmental influences on obesity include food intake and degree of physical activity. Overeating relative to energy needs is a component of obesity development. However, from studies with experimental animals it is clear that many animals that develop obesity are energetically more efficient than lean animals; that is, for a given amount of food, the obesity-prone animals deposit more fat than do the obesity-resistant animals. In fact, when genetically obese rodents are not allowed to overeat from birth, they are still considerably fatter than their lean brothers and sisters. The study of food intake in humans is confounded by the fact that some obese individuals under-report the amount of food they eat. The composition of the diet can also influence obesity. Overweight individuals have been shown to consume more high-fat foods than normal-weight individuals.

The amount of energy that an individual expends will also influence the development of obesity. Increased level of activity is associated with leanness. Other than the energy deficit that occurs with exercise, metabolic changes with training also impact fat utilization and storage. Trained individuals have an increased lipolytic capacity compared to sedentary persons. Both basal and catecholamine-stimulated lipolysis are higher in fat cells from trained individuals. In rats that are obesity-prone, prior to the onset of obesity, catecholamine-stimulated lipolysis is lower in their fat cells than in fat cells from obesity-resistant rats. An important benefit of exercise during weight loss is that it results in preservation of fat-free mass and allows fat loss that is equivalent to or greater than weight loss.

Several physiological factors may be involved in the development of obesity. These include altered adipose tissue metabolism, hormonal changes, and changes at sites in the brain that control satiety, particularly in the hypothalamus. There may be some kind of abnormal signal that affects adipose tissue metabolism and alters fuel partitioning, directing increased storage in adipose tissue instead of use in muscle. This abnormal signal has not been identified. However, lipoprotein lipase has been found to be increased in obesity, and this enzyme can increase the storage of triglycerides in adipose tissue. Hormonal changes that may affect obesity include hyperinsulinemia and changes in pituitary or adrenal function. Hormonal changes during pregnancy promote fat deposition. If weight gain is excessive, it can result in lifelong obesity. The role of psychological variables in the development of obesity is difficult to define. There is no unifying theme.

Some obese individuals have eating disorders. Other obese individuals may eat in response to stress or depression. Still other obese individuals may eat large meals or may eat rapidly. It has also been suggested that some obese individuals may be restrained eaters, and when there is a break in their usual routine, they respond by excessive eating. Although a number of mechanisms have been identified for the development of obesities, the exact picture is far from clear. For many individuals, there may be an underlying biological defect. When this individual comes into contact with a plentiful, good-tasting, high-fat food in an environment that promotes inactivity, obesity results. Also important is the fact that while many people may lose weight, there is little success in keeping the weight off. The reasons for this recidivism and possible solutions are the focus of current research.

Acute Mountain Sickness (AMS)

Acute mountain sickness (AMS) is characterized by a constellation of symptoms. Headache is the main symptom. Nausea, vomiting, dyspnea (shortness of breath), and insomnia are other common symptoms. The traveler at altitude can also experience impaired cognition and balance. Onset of symptoms typically occurs within hours to three days after arrival at altitude. These symptoms tend to resolve after several days but can persist for up to two weeks. They can be the harbinger of the fatal conditions, high-altitude cerebral edema and high-altitude pulmonary edema. At intermediate altitudes, 1,500-3,000 meters, up to 25% of unacclimatized travelers may experience AMS. People with serious lung, heart and blood diseases are more likely to develop AMS. Healthy young adults who participate in vigorous activity upon arrival at altitude are also at great risk for AMS. Individuals with a prior history of AMS and who live at low elevations are especially susceptible. Those who travel rapidly to altitude, as is common with air travel, are also at greater risk for AMS.

Physiologic Effects of Acclimatization and Exercise

Heart

Studies have been conflicting regarding the impact of

increasing altitude on cardiac output and contractility. Laboratory studies using hypobaric chambers to duplicate the effects of altitudes of 4,000 to 8,000 meters have shown a diminished cardiac output at maximal exercise. Other laboratory studies have shown an unchanged or improved cardiac performance at those same altitudes. These studies have shown that, despite a decrease in blood volume and reduced ventricular filling pressure commonly seen at altitude, cardiac output is maintained. Furthermore, an increase in cardiac output is seen at rest and at exercise when compared to the same activities at sea level. This increase is related to an increased sympathetic nervous activity, as demonstrated by increased blood norepinephrine concentration.

On initial exposure to altitudes heart rate increases for a given intensity of exercise, but later the maximal heart rate declines. This decline may be due to altitude-induced increase in activity of the parasympathetic system. The decrease in maximal heart rate may be a beneficial adaptation to limit oxygen consumption.

Lungs

An individual's initial response to the lowered oxygen tension at altitude is to increase ventilation, by increasing the rate and volume of breaths. This phenomenon, the hypoxic ventilatory response, varies between individuals. Clinical studies have shown that those individuals with a history of AMS have a diminished ventilatory response to simulated altitude exposure, as manifest by lower minute ventilation and higher arterial carbon dioxide, despite low transcutaneous oxygen saturation. In contrast, those who remain asymptomatic upon acute exposure to altitude have a high hypoxic ventilatory response. The mechanism for this process remains unclear. As extremes of altitude are reached, the normal lung faces additional impediments in transferring oxygen to the blood. A non-uniform pulmonary arterial vasoconstriction has been demonstrated by using scintigraphy scanning with radiolabeled particles to evaluate the relationship of lung ventilation with pulmonary perfusion. This effect becomes apparent at 3,000 meters. Increasing exercise at this same altitude is also associated with an increasing limitation for the diffusion of oxygen across the alveolar-capillary membrane. At an elevation of 3,900 meters, the unacclimatized individual consumes more oxygen with the increased work of breathing than is gained by that additional ventilation.

There are clear pulmonary conditioning benefits from exercise at intermediate altitude. A greater metabolic efficiency is suggested by a 20% reduction in an individual's oxygen utilization with the same maximal exercise upon return to sea level after intermediate altitude conditioning. Hemoglobin saturation is achieved with lower partial pressures of oxygen and blood levels of 2,3-diphosphoglycerate are elevated after intermediate altitude conditioning. The ability of hemoglobin to carry oxygen to the tissues is further enhanced by the increase in the number of red blood cells.

Muscle

Conditioning at intermediate altitudes results in increased buffering capacity of muscle, increased capillary supply to muscle, and a substantial improvement in aerobic capacity. At extreme altitudes (over 5,000 meters) there is a progressive decrease in muscle fiber size and oxidative enzyme activity. Anaerobic capacity is usually unaltered until altitude exceeds 5,500 meters.

Sleep

Despite fatigue, travelers to altitude often have unrestful sleep because of diminished stage-3, stage-4, and rapid eye-movement sleep. In addition to a diminished quality of sleep, many individuals exhibit periodic breathing at intermediate altitudes, and all do at altitudes over 6,300 meters. Periodic breathing, waxing and waning respirations with periods of apnea, interferes with the already suboptimal arterial oxygenation in the hypobaric environment to produce cycles of even more profound arterial oxygen desaturation. Periodic breathing occurs during 24% of all sleep at 2,440 meters. Lastly, sleep at altitude is characterized by frequent wakening. All of these produce an unsatisfying sleep and contribute to daytime fatigue. As with the other symptoms of AMS at intermediate altitude, sleep can be expected to return to normal with acclimatization. Sleep at very high altitude will remain persistently disturbed.

Fluids/Dehydration

A diuresis takes place with loss of water and sodium during the body's attempt to acclimatize to altitude. This places the individual at risk for dehydration, especially when the individual is involved in maximal exercise. This diuresis is a component of a successful adaptation to altitude. Acute mountain sickness, an unsuccessful adaptation, is characterized by a diminished diuresis, with fluids that are normally in the plasma volume moving into the cells and interstitium, resulting in facial and extremity edema.

Intermediate altitude conditioning commonly involves exposure to a dry and cool atmosphere. A large amount of body water can be lost that will not be apparent to the exercising traveler. Whether symptoms of AMS are present or not, drinking increased volume of fluids is recommended to prevent dehydration, especially with exercise.

Appetite/Nutrition

Nausea and anorexia are common symptoms of AMS at intermediate altitude. Because extra fluid intake is important to replace the fluid loss from high-altitude diuresis, inability to drink and additional losses from vomiting may worsen and prolong the illness. A high-carbohydrate diet may be beneficial, and a low-salt diet may reduce tissue edema. A liquid carbohydrate diet may be easier to tolerate at first exposure to altitude. Because individuals with low iron stores are unable to increase their red cell mass in acclimatization, the diet should be supplemented with iron for those at risk, particularly menstruating females.

Neurologic/Psychiatric

Headache, ranging from subtle to incapacitating, is often the first and most common symptom of AMS. The pain tends to be bilateral and throbbing in quality. It is worse in the morning hours and is exacerbated by strenuous exercise. Individuals with a history of migraine headaches are more likely to develop the headache of AMS. The headaches may be caused by a benign cerebral vasodilatation in response to hypoxia. Acetaminophen, aspirin or ibuprofen may be used along with rest and fluids to ease the headache. Resolution of the headache occurs with acclimatization to intermediate altitude. At very high altitudes, headache may be the first warning sign of cerebral edema. This potentially fatal complication is rarely seen at intermediate altitudes and is associated with changes in the level of consciousness and disturbances in fine motor control and balance. It is treatable only with rapid descent. At very high altitudes, individuals can experience hostile behavior changes, with thoughts of paranoia, depression, anxiety and obsessive-compulsiveness predominating. Those at intermediate altitudes do not experience any behavior changes consistent with increased aggressiveness. Feelings of diminished vigor, weariness, and increased sleepiness are commonly experienced at intermediate altitudes.

Alcohol, Sedatives, Tobacco

Alcohol can impair the altitude acclimatization process in a variety of ways. Alcohol acts as a diuretic and will exacerbate the dehydration seen at altitude. Alcohol can also impair judgment and depress respiration. Similarly, sedative and hypnotic agents impair the sleep-related respiratory cycle. While they may be used by the uninformed altitude traveler to improve the poor quality of sleep that is commonly experienced, the consequence of their ingestion is the further reduction in arterial oxygen saturation during sleep cycling. Furthermore, the type of sleep induced by alcohol and many of the hypnotic agents is not a satisfying, restful sleep. Tobacco poses a number of long-term threats to the individual. A short-term effect of tobacco exposure on the traveler to altitude is the accumulation of carbon monoxide. This toxic gas is present in tobacco smoke and poisons the binding site of hemoglobin for oxygen. At the cellular level, carbon monoxide prevents the utilization of oxygen in cellular respiration.

Prevention and Treatment of Acute Mountain Sickness

Travelers from low elevations who must compete in athletic events at higher altitudes should be aware that the effects of AMS will seriously impair their performance. Their feeling of well-being and ability to remain fit will be compromised. They must allow adequate time for acclimatization. Their acclimatization will occur more rapidly and with fewer symptoms if several recommendations are followed. A slow ascent to altitude, as can be achieved by driving rather than flying to the destination, is associated with milder symptoms. The rate of ascent should be no more than 300 meters a day when above 3,000 meters. Sojourning for a couple of days at an altitude intermediate between the destination altitude and the home altitude is also associated with milder symptoms. After arrival at the destination altitude, heavy exertion should be avoided during the first two days. The traveler should drink plenty of liquids to maintain hydration and eat a high carbohydrate diet. Tobacco, alcohol, and sedative agents must be avoided. If a slow acclimatization is impossible, several medications have shown promise in the prevention or amelioration of AMS.

Acetazolamide is a carbonic-anhydrase inhibitor, which creates a metabolic acidosis due to a renal loss of bicarbonate and an inhibition of red blood cell enzymes with a retention of carbon dioxide. If acetazolamide is taken daily, starting three days before reaching altitude, more than just the overt symptoms of AMS are reduced. The periodic breathing of sleep is reduced, satisfaction of sleep is increased, exercise performance is improved, and higher altitudes can be tolerated. Dexamethasone is a catabolic steroid that is effective in reducing vasogenic cerebral edema. It has been found to reduce the symptoms of AMS with exposure to very high altitudes. Nifedipine, a calcium-channel blocker, may prevent the pulmonary problems seen at very high altitudes. The usefulness of these two agents with intermediate altitude exposure is unclear.

At intermediate altitudes, AMS is very unlikely to progress to the severe illness seen at very high elevations. If serious illness does occur, descent remains the only definitive intervention. A dramatic improvement can occur with as little as a 300-meter descent. The natural history of intermediate altitude AMS is improvement within 3-5 days. If the symptoms are very uncomfortable, or if they interfere with normal activities, improvement can occur with the administration of supplemental oxygen, oral or intravenous rehydration, rest, and treatment with either acetazolamide or dexamethasone.

Anabolic-Androgenic Steroids

Anabolic steroids are drugs that resemble androgenic hormones (sometimes called male hormones) such as testosterone. Athletes consume them in the hope of gaining weight, strength, power, speed, endurance, and aggressiveness. They are widely used by athletes involved in such sports as track and field (mostly the throwing events), weight lifting, and American football. However, in spite of their tremendous popularity, their effectiveness is controversial. The research literature is divided on whether anabolic steroids enhance physical performance. Yet, almost all athletes who consume these substances acclaim their beneficial effects. Many athletes feel that they would not have been as successful without them. There are several possible reasons for the large differences between experimental findings and empirical observations. An incredible mystique has arisen around these substances, providing fertile ground for the placebo effect. The use of anabolic steroids in the "real world" is considerably different from that in rigidly controlled, double-blind experiments (in a double blind study, neither the subject nor experimenter knows who is taking the drug). Most studies have not used the same drug dosage used by athletes. Institutional safeguards prohibit administration of high dosages of possibly dangerous substances to human subjects. Subjects in research experiments seldom resemble accomplished weight-trained athletes. Under these conditions, we must assess the results of sound research studies, as well as clinical and empirical field observations, in order to obtain a realistic profile of the use, effects on performance, and side effects of these substances.

Male hormones, principally testosterone, are partially responsible for the tremendous developmental changes that occur during puberty and adolescence. Male hormones have androgenic and anabolic effects. Androgenic effects are changes in primary and secondary sexual characteristics. These include enlargement of the penis and testes, voice changes, hair growth on the face, axilla, and genital areas, and increased aggressiveness. The anabolic effects of androgens include accelerated growth of muscle, bone, and red blood cells, and enhanced neural conduction. Anabolic steroids have been manufactured to enhance the anabolic properties (tissue building) of the androgens and minimize the androgenic (sex-linked) properties. However, no steroid has eliminated the androgenic effects because the so-called androgenic effects are really anabolic effects in sex-linked tissues. The effects of male hormones on accessory sex glands, genital hair growth, and oiliness of the skin are anabolic processes in those tissues. The steroids with the most potent anabolic effect are also those with the greatest androgenic effect.

Steroid Receptors

Steroid hormones work by stimulation of receptor molecules in muscle cells, which activate specific genes to produce proteins. They also affect the activation rate of enzyme systems involved in protein metabolism, thus enhancing protein synthesis and inhibiting protein degradation (called an anti-catabolic effect).

Heavy resistance training seems to be necessary for anabolic steroids to exert any beneficial effect on physical performance. Most research studies that have demonstrated improved performance with anabolic steroids used experienced weight lifters who were capable of training with heavier weights and producing relatively greater muscle tension during exercise than novice subjects. The effectiveness of anabolic steroids is dependent upon unbound receptor sites in muscle. Intense strength training may increase the number of unbound receptor sites. This would increase the effectiveness of anabolic steroids.

Anti-Catabolic Effects Of Anabolic Steroids

Many athletes have said that anabolic steroids help them train harder and recover faster. They also said that they had difficulty making progress (or even holding onto the gains) when they were off the drugs. Anabolic steroids may have an anti-catabolic effect. This means that the drugs may prevent muscle catabolism that often accompanies intense exercise training. Presently, this hypothesis has not been fully proven. Anabolic steroids may block the effects of hormones such as cortisol involved in tissue breakdown during and after exercise. Anabolic steroids may prevent tissue from breaking down following of an intense work-out. This would speed recovery. Cortisol and related hormones, secreted by the adrenal cortex, also has receptor sites within skeletal muscle cells. Cortisol causes protein breakdown and is secreted during exercise to enhance the use of proteins for fuel and to suppress inflammation that accompanies tissue injury. Anabolic steroids may block the binding of cortisol to its receptor sites, which would prevent muscle breakdown and enhances recovery. While this is beneficial while the athlete is taking the drug, the effect backfires when he stops taking it.

Hormonal adaptations occur in response to the abnormal amount of male hormone present in the athlete's body. Cortisol receptor sites and cortisol secretion from the adrenal cortex increase. Anabolic steroid use decreases testosterone secretion. People who stop taking steroids are also hampered with less male hormone than usual during the "off" periods. The catabolic effects of cortisol are enhanced when the athlete stops taking the drugs and strength and muscle size are lost at a rapid rate.

The rebound effect of cortisol and its receptors presents people who use anabolic steroids with several serious problems:

(1) psychological addiction is more probable because they become dependent on the drugs. This is because they tend to lose strength and size rapidly when off steroids. To stave off deconditioning, athletes may want to take the drugs for long periods of time to prevent falling behind.

(2) Long-term administration increases the chance of serious side-effects.

(3) Cortisol suppresses the immune system. This makes steroid users more prone to diseases, such as cold and flu, during the period immediately following steroid administration.

Psychological Effects

Some researchers have speculated that the real effect of anabolic steroids is the creation of a "psychosomatic state" characterized by sensations of well being, euphoria, increased aggressiveness and tolerance to stress, allowing the athlete to train harder. Such a psychosomatic state would be more beneficial to experienced weight lifters who have developed the motor skills to exert maximal force during strength training. Diets high in protein and calories may also be important in maximizing the effectiveness of anabolic steroids.

Anabolic Steroids and Performance

The effects of anabolic steroids on physical performance

are unclear. Well controlled, double blind studies have rendered conflicting results. In studies showing beneficial effects, body weight increased by an average of about four pounds, lean body weight by about six pounds (fat loss accounts for the discrepancy between gains in lean mass and body weight), bench press increased by about 15 pounds, and squats by about 30 pounds (these values represent the average gains for all studies showing a beneficial effect). Almost all studies have failed to demonstrate a beneficial effect on maximal oxygen consumption or endurance capacity. Anabolic steroid studies have typically lasted six to eight weeks and have usually used relatively untrained subjects.

Most changes in strength during the early part of training are neural: increased strength is mainly due to an improved ability to recruit motor units. Anabolic steroids affect processes associated with protein synthesis in muscle. Studies lasting six weeks (typical study length) would largely reflect neural changes and could easily miss the cellular effects of the drugs.

The gains made by athletes in uncontrolled observations have been much more impressive. Weight gains of thirty or forty pounds, coupled with thirty percent increases in strength, are not unusual. Such case studies lack credibility because of the absence of scientific controls. However, it would be foolish to completely disregard such observations because the "subjects" have been highly trained and motivated athletes.Please see the articles on pharmacology of sport and sports medicine in the countries of the former Soviet Union for more information on anabolic steroids.

Tai chi: A Traditional Chinese Exercise

Tai chi, a traditional Chinese exercise, has been practiced for centuries in China by the elderly and young to attain agility, balance, and posture control. Its beneficial effects on health have been observed, and the maintenance of balance control in older people in particular has drawn increasing attention from scientific researchers. A number of cross sectional and longitudinal studies have provided positive evidence that tai chi practitioners not only have better cardiorespiratory function, but also perform better in balance control, flexibility, and muscle strength tests.

Although many studies have confirmed the effects of tai chi exercise on balance control for the elderly, little effort has been devoted to determining the underlying mechanism. Postural equilibrium needs proprioceptive acuity and precise neuromuscular control. Proprioception is the afferent information that contributes to conscious sensation (muscle sense), total posture (postural equilibrium), and segmental posture (joint stability).

Many studies have indicated that proprioception diminishes with age. Gerontologists have postulated that impaired proprioception makes it difficult for older people to detect changes in body position until it is too late for compensatory behaviour to prevent falls. Indeed, some studies have shown that diminished proprioception is a major contributing factor to falls in the elderly. It is very important for old people to retain this ability.

One strategy to reduce the incidence of poor proprioception and falls with aging may be regular physical activity.Exercise can help to improve a number of sensorimotor systems that contribute to stability. However, different forms of exercise may have different effects on postural equilibrium. Tai chi exercise requires continuous, slow movement with small to large expressions of motion, the shift of body weight from unilateral to bilateral, and circular movements of the trunk and extremities, involving both isometric and isotonic contractions.

All forms of tai chi emphasise conscious awareness of body position and movement, which seem to contain the characteristics of proprioceptive exercise. Therefore does tai chi exercise have particular benefits for old people's proprioception? 12 week tai chi programme could increase participants' shoulder kinaesthetic sense at 60°. However, the mean (SD) age of the subjects was 30.4 (4.3) years, and the investigators did not consider the principal joint systems of the lower extremity (ankle, knee, and hip) involved in postural control. This study was therefore designed to investigate the proprioception of ankle and knee joints in elderly long term tai chi practitioners, long term swimmers/runners, and sedentary controls.

The purpose was to assess whether long term tai chi practice could improve proprioception and whether the effect of tai chi on proprioception was more evident than other common activities in the elderly. Such information would help to explain the mechanism whereby tai chi exercise improves balance.

Methods

By means of a questionnaire with a complementary interview about their physical and sporting activities, 68 old people were recruited to the study. They were predominantly healthy with no history of major cardiovascular, pulmonary, metabolic, musculoskeletal, or neurological diseases. Twenty one subjects had regularly practiced tai chi for approximately 1.5 hours a day over the previous four years or more (TC group). Twenty subjects had swum and/or run for at least one hour a day for four or more years (S/R group).

The subjects in the TC and S/R groups had not done any other regular physical activity in the previous five years. Twenty seven subjects had not engaged in any regular exercise for more than four years (control group). No significant difference was noted in sex, age, height, and weight across the three groups (table 1). Each subject gave written informed consent before participation. The study was approved by the local medical ethics committee.

Measurement procedures

Joint kinaesthesis is the sensation of joint movement; it is an important technique used to evaluate proprioception. Kinaesthesis is usually determined by establishing the threshold at which passive motion is detected, an assessment of the ability to detect relatively slow passive joint motion. We used it to assess knee and ankle joint proprioception. Testing was performed in a well lit and well ventilated room. The room was sound attenuated and isolated so as to reduce any auditory or visual interference that might distract the participants. After their weight and height had been measured, each subject participated in two separate data collection sessions: measurement of ankle joint kinaesthesis and, after a brief rest period, measurement of knee joint kinaesthesis.

Ankle joint kinaesthesis test

The device is also equipped with a hanging scale and a fixed pulley supported by a trestle, which is outside of the device. A thigh cuff attached to the lower end of the scale is wrapped around the lower thigh of the subject. By adjustment of the length of the cuff, the extremity is lifted by the scale, and its weight is recorded when the subject fully relaxes the thigh. The thigh cuff is then attached to one end of the rope around the pulley and the other end is hung with weights.

The extremity can then be adjusted to where the foot is in contact with the platform. By adding or reducing the weights, the investigator can standardise the weight of the lower extremity resting on the platform during testing. For data collection, each subject was seated on an adjustable chair and his or her dominant foot was placed on the platform so that the axis of the apparatus coincided with the plantar dorsiflexion axis of the ankle joint. The hip, knee, and ankle were positioned at 90°. To standardise the sensory cues from the contact between the instrument and the plantar surface of the foot, 50% of the lower extremity weight was rested on the platform by the use of the thigh cuff suspension system.

During testing, subjects kept their eyes closed and wore headphones with music playing to eliminate visual and auditory stimuli from the testing apparatus. Each test movement began with the foot placed on the horizontal platform-that is, the starting position was 0°. The subjects were instructed to concentrate on their foot and to press the hand switch when they could sense motion and identify the direction of the movement. After two practice trials had been performed, the motor was engaged to rotate the foot into dorsiflexion or plantarflexion at a random time interval between two and ten seconds after subject instruction. The researcher recorded the rotation angles of the platform and the direction of movements as passive motion sense. At least six randomised trials were conducted: three for plantarflexion, three for dorsiflexion. The mean values of the three angles sensed in one direction were calculated.

Table 1

Characteristics of elderly tai chi practitioners (TC group), swimmers/runners (S/R group), and sedentary controls (Control group)

	Group Age (years)	*Height (cm)*	*Weight (kg)*
TC (n = 21, 12M, 9F)	66.1 (5.2)	163.6 (7.9)	64.8 (9.9)
S/R (n = 20, 12M, 8F)	65.4 (3.0)	164.1 (8.6)	66.5 (12.4)
Control (n = 27, 15M, 12F)	65.6 (3.9)	163.9 (7.8)	68.5 (10.9)

Knee joint kinaesthesis test

The subjects wore shorts to negate any extraneous skin sensation from clothing at the knee area. They sat in an adjustable chair with legs hanging freely over the edge of the seat 5 cm proximal to the popliteal fossa. A custom made inflatable cuff was fitted above the knee joint and inflated to 20 mm Hg to neutralise cutaneous sensation. The axis of rotation of the knee joint was aligned with the axis of rotation of the frame. Then the researcher placed the lower part of the shank of the subject on the frame. An ankle inflatable cuff was applied and inflated to 20 mm Hg to reduce multisensory afferent discharge at the shank-machine interface. To further reduce unwanted sensory input, the subjects kept their eyes closed and wore headphones with music playing to eliminate the sight and sound of the apparatus. The starting position of each trial was 45°of knee flexion as measured by an electrogoniometer. Subjects were told that their legs could move in a flexed or extended direction beginning at a random delay of 2-10 seconds after the examiner signalled the start of the test. Once the subject detected motion of the leg, he or she pressed a hand held stop button and confirmed the direction of the motion. The rotation angles of the frame were defined as the threshold of detection for the knee joint. Mean values of three trials in one direction were used for analysis.

All variables are presented as mean (SD). Values for passive motion sense of ankle and knee joint in different directions were respectively compared using paired *t* test in each group. Because there were no significant differences between the directions of ankle movement, plantarflexion, and dorsiflexion, data were averaged to produce ankle kinaesthesis. One way analysis of variance was used to estimate significant differences among groups. Post hoc Scheffe tests were performed when necessary to isolate the differences, and p(0.05 was considered significant.

Ankle joint kinaesthesis

Ankle joint kinaesthesis differed significantly among the three groups ($p = 0.001$). Movements of 1.21 (0.33)°were perceived in the TC group, 1.78 (0.82)°in the S/R group, and 1.95 (0.66)°in the sedentary control group. The post hoc test showed that the TC group could detect a significantly smaller amount of motion than the control group (p = 0.001) and S/ R group (p = 0.022), while no significant difference was found between the S/R group and sedentary control group (p = 0.701).

Knee joint kinaesthesis

The threshold for detection of passive motion was significantly different in extension and flexion for each group; the knees were more sensitive to a flexion arc than to an extension arc. One way analysis of variance indicated significant differences in passive motion sense in knee flexion across the three groups (p = 0.025). Further analysis showed that the TC group had a significantly lower mean threshold for detection of passive motion than the subjects in the control group (p = 0.026). There were no significant differences between the S/R group and control group (p = 0.312), or between the TC group and S/R group (p = 0.533). For knee extension, no significant difference was found among the three groups (p = 0.597).

Although many studies have indicated that adoption of regular physical activity can attenuate the age related decline in many physiological systems, few have examined the effects of exercise on proprioception of old people, especially the effects of different kinds of exercise. The study shows that long term tai chi practitioners not only have better ankle and knee joint kinaesthesis than sedentary controls but also their ankle joint kinaesthesis is better than regular swimmers/ runners. Furthermore, the latter did not perform any better in ankle and knee joint kinaesthesis tests than their sedentary counterparts. The postural control system operates as a control circuit between the sensory sources, central nervous system, and the musculoskeletal system. Proprioceptors and visual and vestibular centres contribute afferent information to the central nervous system on body position and balance. Colledge and his colleagues studied the relative contributions to balance of vision, proprioception, and the vestibular system in different age groups. They found all age groups were more dependent on proprioception than on vision for the maintenance of balance. Thus proprioception may greatly influence postural stability, and a decline in proprioception with aging could be associated with the increased propensity of elderly people to fall.8 The considerable benefits of tai chi exercise on proprioception may have significance for old people in maintaining balance. Training has been widely reported to be one of the best ways to improve balance in the elderly. However, different kinds of exercise have been shown to have different effects on balance. Gauchard et al chose yoga and soft gymnastics as proprioceptive exercise, which consist of slow movements performed sequentially under different postural conditions; they compared the effects of proprioceptive exercise, bioenergetic physical activities (swimming, cycling, or jogging), and no exercise on postural control in elderly people.

The results indicate that muscular strength was significantly increased in the bioenergetic exercise group, but proprioceptive exercise appeared to have the greatest effect on balance control. The authors pointed out that the ritual motions of tai chi are also proprioceptive exercise. From our results showing that elderly tai chi practitioners have improved proprioception, we suggest that maintaining, or delaying the decline, in proprioception is closely associated with tai chi exercise improving balance control in old people.

Tai chi exercise is a series of individual graceful movements in a slow, continuous, circular pattern. In performing tai chi, awareness of movement sequencing starts from the feet, ankles, and legs, and the strong thigh muscles are used to concentrate the movement through and around the turning of the hips and waist, with the latter acting as the axis around which all body movements are executed.

The movements of tai chi are gracefully fluent and consummately precise because specificity of joint angles and body position is of critical importance in accurately and correctly performing each form. Acute awareness of body position and movement is demanded by the nature of the activity. Thus it is logical that the practice of tai chi has benefits for proprioception, which is confirmed by our study.

Swimming and running are two of the most common exercises practiced by elderly people; they are excellent forms of aerobic exercise, and provide good training stimuli for cardiopulmonary function and muscle strength. Compared with tai chi, swimming and running involve cyclic repetitive actions. Awareness of joint position and movement is not emphasised during these exercise forms. In addition, most elderly people exercise only to enhance health and for recreation; they usually do not pay much attention to joint position and angles during exercise, unless such awareness is required in certain forms of exercise, such as tai chi. This may help to explain why the swimmers/runners did not have better scores for knee and ankle kinaesthesis in this study. It is of particular interest that the effects of tai chi on proprioception were different in the knee and ankle joints.

The effect on ankle joint kinaesthesis was more prominent than on knee joint kinaesthesis. The passive motion sense of the ankle joint in the TC group was significantly better than in both the sedentary control group and the S/R group. However, for the knee joint, tai chi exercise only produced a better effect than in the sedentary control group. These results may be attributable to the characteristics of tai chi movements. The old tai chi proverb states, "When performing tai chi, the feet act as roots". Although almost all tai chi forms are performed in a semi-squat position, which enhances the loading of the muscles and motion ranges of the knee joints, the continuous transformation of different postures and steps cause more changes in ankle joint movements, such as turning the toes outward or inward and raising or lowering the toes. Moreover, while making a stride, foot placement is slow and deliberate. These movements may help to retain the sensitivity of proprioceptors located in the joint capsules, ligaments, tendons, and muscles. Ankle proprioception is very important for the elderly to maintain proper postural control.

Many studies have indicated that the movement pattern for postural correction in elderly adults is different from that of young adults. The elderly rely more on hip movements, while young people rely on ankle movements to control postural stability. A decline in somatosensory information from the feet is a major factor in this pattern change with age. Therefore the considerable impact of tai chi practice on ankle proprioception is of great benefit in the retention of balance control in old people.

The decline in proprioception with age may be an important contributing factor to falls in the elderly, and this may be influenced by regular physical activity. This study shows that, compared with other common activities, long term tai chi exercise may have more benefit in retaining proprioception of the ankle and knee joints, which may be valuable for maintaining balance control in the elderly.

Sports Medicine

Sports Medicine is the field of medicine concerned with injuries sustained in athletic endeavors, including their prevention, diagnosis, and treatment. The purpose of injury prevention and treatment is to maintain optimal health and maximize peak performance. Traditionally, sports medicine was the sole domain of the team doctor, who worked mostly with college, professional, and Olympic athletes.

Today, however, the sports medicine team is comprised of many disciplines including, for example, athletic training, biomechanics, exercise physiology, and nutrition. Sports medicine specialists also work with non-professional athletes and those participating in various recreational activities, for example children involved in youth sports or older adults training for foot races. Exercise Science is the study of movement and the associated functional responses and adaptations. In this context, an exercise scientist must understand the scientific basis underlying exercise-induced physiological responses. The field of exercise science involves a range of disciplines similar to those in sports medicine; consequently, it is common for exercise science professionals to work in sports medicine facilities.

The field of exercise science, however, is typically much broader than sports medicine, ranging from the study of how organ systems work at the cellular level when confronted with disease, to improving the biomechanical efficiency of an employee working on an assembly line. Strict categorizing of a specific discipline (for example, exercise physiologist, dietitian, biomechanist) to either sports medicine or exercise science is difficult. It simply depends on the emphasis and application of the setting in which one works. What is important to understand is that many different disciplines comprise what is called sports medicine and exercise science. And they work together as a team in order to understand and ultimately improve the health and performance of the whole individual. Without this multidisciplinary approach to the whole person, the end result tends to be less than optimal. A rigorous training program, for example, may have little impact on the health or performance of an individual if nutritional considerations are neglected.

Aerobics/group exercise instructor

An aerobics instructor leads exercise sessions for a group of participants. The group may be heterogeneous, including individuals with different fitness levels, medical concerns and ages, or homogeneous, with individuals who have similar characteristics such as arthritis, frail and elderly, or pregnancy. Examples of group exercise instruction include land- or water-based dance/step aerobics, chair aerobics, and cycling. Aerobics instructors can be employed in a variety of settings including commercial fitness centers, employee fitness programs, or hospitals. Minimal requirements are an undergraduate degree and some type of recognized certification, such as that from the American College of Sports Medicine.

Athletic Trainer

Athletic trainers work with team physicians, exercise physiologists, physical therapists and coaches in the care and prevention of illness and injury related to sports and exercise. An undergraduate degree from an accredited program by the Commission on Accreditation of Allied Health Education Programs (CAAHEP) is required to sit for the National Athletic Trainers' Association (NATA) certification examination beginning in the year 2004. In most states licensure is required. One of the requirements for licensure is to successfully pass the NATA certification examination. Athletic trainers typically work with athletes at the high school, college, or professional level. They might also be employed in sports medicine clinics.

Biomechanist

Biomechanics is the study and explanation of the laws of physics as applied to physical activity, exercise and sport. Biomechanics can be used to explain how muscles, bones, and joints are injured under certain conditions and to improve performance using motion analysis techniques. Biomechanists are typically employed in research settings and clinical sites, but future growth appears to be in industrial ergonomic settings. Minimal requirement is a master's degree.

Cardiopulmonary Rehabilitation Specialist

This exercise specialist provides both immediate and longterm guidance for the physical rehabilitation of individuals who have one or more cardiac or pulmonary-related conditions or diseases, such as heart attack, heart surgery, or emphysema. A major component of this physical rehabilitation is to administer and supervise exercise testing and training sessions. Hospitals hire exercise specialists and require at least an undergraduate degree. However, opportunities for employment improve with an advanced degree and some type of recognized certification, such as that by the American College of Sports Medicine.

Dietitian/Sports Nutritionist

Dietetics is the study of nutrient intake and how foods are digested and metabolized in order to provide the necessary energy to fuel muscular activity. Dietitians also study dietary patterns in order to maximize performance and to prevent disease and improve health. To become a registered dietitian, you must complete an undergraduate degree in dietetics, complete a nine-month American Dietetics Association (ADA) approved internship and pass the ADA certification examination. Dietitians can be employed in a variety of settings including hospitals, clinics, school systems, and public health facilities.

Employee Fitness Director

Employee fitness programs are common in the workplace, especially in large companies. Along with conducting exercise programs, the exercise scientist may also be trained as a wellness specialist to provide broad-based health promotion and wellness education programs. These may include stress management and nutrition education programs. Traditionally, workplace exercise programs have been for healthy individuals only. However, to reduce health care costs, employee fitness centers are becoming more clinically based in terms of exercise training all employees, including those with cardiac, pulmonary or musculoskeletal problems. At least an undergraduate degree is required. It is also recommended to obtain a recognized certification, such as that by the American College of Sports Medicine.

Exercise Physiologist

An exercise physiologist studies the acute and chronic physiological responses and adaptations resulting from physical activity. They can apply this knowledge to improve or maintain health, fitness or performance. Traditionally, exercise physiologists worked and studied only with athletes to improve performance. Today, however, exercise physiologists also work and study in commercial, clinical, and workplace settings to increase health, fitness, and quality of life of the general population. For example, an exercise physiologist may work as a cardiopulmonary rehabilitation specialist, a personal trainer, or direct an employee fitness program. At least an undergraduate degree is required.

Medical Physician

A medical physician is highly trained in the art and science of the diagnosis and treatment of disease and the maintenance of health. Medical schools require a minimum of four years after a basic college degree. Beyond medical school there are many specialties to choose from in order to be part of a sports medicine or exercise science team.

Such specialties might include primary care sports medicine, orthopedic surgery, or cardiology. Each specialty has from three to five years of intern and residency training and perhaps an additional one to two years of fellowship training. Most medical doctors are employed in clinics or hospitals.

Occupational Physiologist

Occupational physiologists work with many different professionals to improve the performance of workers by enhancing their health and occupational abilities, preventing or rehabilitating workplace injuries, and redesigning the work environment to fit the worker. They may also develop and administer pre-employment physical capacity tests to determine if the worker is fit to perform the job. An advanced degree beyond the undergraduate level is typically required, and it is helpful to be certified by the Board of Certification in Professional Ergonomics.

Personal Trainer

A personal trainer typically works oneon-one with an individual and is generally paid by the hour or exercise session. The exercise session can take place at the client's home, the trainer's place of employment or business, or at a thirdparty fitness facility. In reality, all exercise scientists who work with exercising adults are personal trainers because of the individual exercise prescription that is given to each client based upon their health status, goals, and the like. At least an undergraduate degree and recognized certification, such as that by the American College of Sports Medicine, is recommended.

Physical/Occupational Therapist

A physical therapist helps people recover from injuries or diseases of the muscles, joints, nerves or bones. An occupational therapist works more with fine motor skills and dexterity. Both therapists use various physical modalities and exercise, focusing on movement dysfunction. There are many areas of specialization in physical therapy including cardiopulmonary rehabilitation, sports medicine and biomechanics. Most physical and occupational therapy schools require two to three years after a four-year undergraduate degree. Following formal training one must pass a national examination to become a licensed physical or occupational therapist. Most employment opportunities are in hospitals and clinics.

Researcher

Researchers conduct studies from either a basic or applied scientist's perspective. Basic researchers usually conduct studies with a focus on the cellular and molecular levels, such as how organ systems work, adapts or respond to various factors. Sometimes this is referred to as bench research, especially if animal models are used. Applied researchers usually conduct studies with a focus on more practical questions that appear to be more applicable for immediate use, such as ways to increase athletic performance or how to improve health and reduce disease. Either career requires getting a terminal degree, such as a Ph.D., which involves at least four to five years beyond the undergraduate level. Most researchers are employed in universities and hospitals.

Strength (Sport) and conditioning coach

Sports teams at the high school, college and professional level employ strength and conditioning coaches. Their role is to develop and supervise specific conditioning programs to increase athletic performance such as speed, agility, strength, endurance, flexibility and power. Positions usually require a master's degree and certification by the National Strength and Conditioning Association.

Teacher

Teachers can be employed at the elementary through college level. If you desire to teach physical education or coach at the elementary or secondary level, an undergraduate degree is required, and you must be certified by the state in which you teach. With a master's degree you may be able to teach at a college or university, especially if coupled with practical experience. However, these opportunities are limited. In higher education, it is customary to hire those with a terminal degree, such as a Ph.D., which is four to five years beyond the undergraduate level. Teachers at the college or university level often conduct research. As you can tell from this partial list there is a diversity of career and job opportunities, fields of study, and specialty areas in sports medicine and exercise science. What may be of importance to you is that most undergraduate degrees in the sports medicine or exercise science field require a strong background in the basic sciences. This provides a strong foundation to meet the requirements for an advanced degree or for a professional school (for example, to become a physician assistant or physical therapist). Check with schools that interest you to identify the specific requirements for admission to these type of advanced or professional-degree programs.

Sports medicine and exercise science are exciting and growing career paths. If you are interested in pursuing a career in these areas, the best advice is to obtain as much information as you can about the profession.

9

Sports and Tissue Damage

Within the human spinal canal the spinal cord extends from the base of the brain to the conus medallaris usually at the level of the L1/L2 vertebrae when the nerve roots become the cauda equina. The spinal cord is a soft, pliable mass of nerve fibres and cells supported by glial tissue and enmeshed in small blood vessels. The cord contains myelinated 'long' tracts and interconnecting fibres described as the 'white matter' surrounding the central 'grey matter' comprising mostly unmyelinated nerve fibres with supporting glial tissue and a very intense small blood vessel network. Blood flow to the spinal cord is mainly provided to the anterior tow-thirds of the cord by the anterior spinal artery which arises from two branches of each vertebral artery over the medulla and runs superficially in the anterior sulcus to eventually synapse around the lower end of the spinal cord with the descending branches of the posterior spinal arteries which arise from the posterior inferior cerebellar arteries. Posterior spinal arteries provide blood flow to the posterior third of the spinal cord.

These small spinal arteries require additional assistance from the major supplementary arterial supply usually at two levels of the spinal cord (T1 and T11), from the corresponding intercostal arteries. Nerve fibres in the posterior columns of white matter are essentially travelling cephalward and are uncrossed until higher in the central nervous system carrying sensory modalities for proprioception, vibration, some touch and appreciation of moderate degrees of temperature variation. Tracts in the anterior column of white matter are mainly travelling caudalward to synapse either directly with anterior horn cells or with other interneuronal pathways. In the lateral column there is a mix of fibres going 'upwards and downwards'.

The lateral column contains the lateral cortico-spinal pathway (pyramidal pathway) for control of motor power and anteriorly is the main tract for pain (spino-thalamic) which are mostly crossed fibres. In the cervical spinal cord the nerves in this tract have a laminated arrangement with the most distant fibres travelling towards the distal end of the body (sacral) and the cervical travelling more central within the tract. Anteriorly to the pain pathway is the main pathway for temperature and further anteriorly again is the pathway for touch. Touch appears to be transmitted in the anterior and posterior columns.

The cortico-spinal pathway also has a layered orientation with those motor fibres destined to synapse with anterior horn cells in the lower spinal cord (lumbo-sacral) travelling in the more superficial layers of the tract in the cervical region. There remains a complex arborisation of synapsing fibres within the spinal cord and many interneuronal pathways are necessary to achieve balanced efferent and afferent activities within the human spinal cord. The spinal cord tends to occupy only 50% of the ligamentum denticulatum and in the intervertebral foramina.

The dura mater is also attached firmly to the base of the skull and at the second fused segment of the sacrum in the adult (filum terminale). There is therefore a lateral attachment of the spinal cord to both sides of the spinal canal. The spinal cord within the dura is a mobile organ which tends to be held more tightly in the flexed position of the spine and in a more relaxed position when the spine is extended. The spinal canal is formed by 26 vertebra, 24 usually being separate from each other but attached with intervening discs, ligaments and muscles.

The coccyx is attached to the lower end of the sacrum and usually comprises 4 small fused vertebrae of a vestigial 'tail'. The sacrum usually consists of 5 vertebra also fused together. The stable spinal column is maintained with a cervical lordotic curve, a thoracic kyphotic curve and a lumbar lordotic curve. There are fixed kyphotic curves in the fused sacrum and coccyx. The spinal vertebral column can be subdivided into the Denis 3 column classification, with an anterior column, which includes the anterior longitudinal spinal ligament, the anterior annulus of the disc and the anterior third of the vertebral body; the middle column under this classification includes the posterior spinal longitudinal ligament, the posterior annulus of the disc and the posterior two thirds of the vertebral body; the posterior column involves the posterior bony arch with the spines, laminae and pedicles, and attached ligaments including supraspinous, interpinous, ligamentum flavum and capsules of the posterior facet joints.

The muscles immediately surrounding the spinal column and attached to the vertebrae are of great importance in maintaining stability of the spinal column. In addition to those muscles which are closely applied to the vertebrae, there is the additional 'wider circle' of muscles which includes the larger spinal muscles, for example, trapezius, latissimus dorsi and the abdominal muscles. Each disc has a firm annulus fibrosus surrounding the nucleus pulposus, which is softer, pliable material and each disc is firmly attached to the adjacent surfaces of the vertebra above and below. The posterior spinal longitudinal ligament is loosely attached to the discs. The annulus fibrosus has a nerve supply from the sinu vertebral nerve of Luschka.

Injury

Damage to the spinal cord can either occur from direct injury to the spinal cord tissue, including nerves, cells and supporting tissue (glia) within the spinal membranes or through injury to the blood vessels essential for cord function. Damage can occur to the anterior spinal artery, posterior spinal arteries and the circumferential arteries which give off radiate branches running into the deeper central regions of the spinal cord. There is also a complex network of very small vessels, particularly within the grey matter which can be injured. There is now evidence to suggest further progressive damage will occur to nerves in the spinal cord within hours of the initial injury due to changes which occur in microvascular tissue within both grey and white matter. The exact nature of these progressive pathological changes has yet to be fully identified. A lack of efficient blood flow to the partly damaged nerve tissue can lead to additional ischaemia and further damage to nerves which may have otherwise survived the initial direct injury.

Damage to the spinal cord is described as 'complete' if laceration or severe bruising has occurred at the level of the lesion. In adults this injury is frequently associated with disturbance of the bony canal following fracture or fracture dislocation. In children there is often no obvious radiological evidence of significant damage to the vertebral column. Less serious injuries are described as 'incomplete' spinal cord injuries, eg. in concussion where the pathological changes are reversible with scattered small areas of haemorrhage in grey and white matter without disruption of the cord structure. Contusion, or bruising, which can be described as being (I) 'mild' where haemorrhages are larger in number and size than in concussion and with some permanent damage to nerve fibres and cells; (II) 'moderate' with increased damage and severe bruising resulting in complete loss of cord function.

The various areas of the spinal cord can be damaged resulting in specific clinical syndromes; eg. the Brown-Sequard syndrome where damage is confined mostly to one half of the spinal cord; the anterior column syndrome where the antero-lateral columns are affected often by damage to the anterior spinal artery; the central cord syndrome where the grey matter is the essentially affected area resulting in central cystic changes an profound loss of anterior columns without significant loss in other areas and this injury produces severe disability with loss of proprioception even though there is usually significant voluntary movement below the level of the lesion.

Bones

Fractures in the vertebral bodies are described as wedge fractures, from flexion and compression injuries; extension fractures are associated with 'shearing' translational injuries; compression fractures is a burst injury to the vertebral body with retropulsion; a slice injury which can occur as a flexion and rotation causing damage to the vertebral body and interspinous and supraspinous ligament between the vertebrae.

Spondylolysis occurs with a defect in the pars interarticularis of the vertebral body. If the defect is bilateral possible shift may occur in the anterior and middle column segments of the spine following separation from the posterior spinal column segment. This is described as spondylolisthesis and identified as grade 1, i.e. 25% of the shift forward of one vertebra in relationship to another, up to greater than 50% of the vertebral displacement (grade 4). Ligaments and joint capsules are usually damaged including the interspinous ligaments, facet joint capsules, posterior longitudinal and anterior longitudinal ligament to allow subluxation of facet joints with the anterior vertebral subluxation. These injuries can be found in fast bowlers, baseball pitchers, gymnasts and weight lifters.

Damage can occur to the intervertebral discs resulting in mild bulging of the annulus, increasing to bulging with tearing of the fibrous annular tissue if more severe. Rupturing of the disc results when the nucleus pulposus herniates through a break in the annular wall frequently impinging on nearby spinal cord, cauda equina or emerging nerve roots.

Damage to specific vertebrae

The C1 and C2 vertebrae (atlas and axis) damage. Fracture of the C1 ring secondary to axial compression can result in a Jefferson type fracture. Rupture of the transverse ligament of the atlas produces instability. Consider potential instability if the atlanto-axial space is greater than 3mms in flexion in the adult and 4mms in a child. Fractures of the odontoid frequently produce pain which radiates posteriorly into the occipital area. The odontoid fractures are divided into type 1 where there is a small segment of the odontoid fractured; type 2 where the base of the odontoid is fractured; and type 3 where the fracture extends from the base of the odontoid into the body of the C2 vertebra. A 'hangman's fracture' (traumatic spondylolisthesis) occurs through the pedicles of C2 following hyperextension of the head and neck.

Damage to muscles, ligaments and tendons

Mild damage to muscles involves over stretch or direct bruising with more severe injury when muscle fibres are torn or disrupted at the insertion of the tendon. The ruptured fibres in the muscle belly will retract and ultimately heal with less elastic scar tissue. The post traumatic inflammatory process can localise at the insertion of muscles, tendons and ligaments near bone and is described as enthesopathic inflammatory process which can lead to calcification. The sites commonly involved are the insertion of the outer layer of the annulus fibrosus into the vertebral body, sometimes causing bony bridges between adjacent vertebrae (syndesmophytes). Injury to musculo-skeletal tissue may highlight previously undiagnosed spondylarthropathies including ankylosing spondylitis, spondylitis associated with psoriasis, enteropathic syndromes, Reiter's disease and arthritis associated with positive 'rheumatoid factor'.

Estosterone and Reproductive Dysfunction

Endurance training can result in dysfunction in the reproductive system of humans. Research within the sports medicine community has primarily focused upon reproductive dysfunction associated with athletic women. Not until recently have studies seriously addressed the question of how exercise training affects the male reproductive system. Research findings in this area have led some investigators to suggest that the effect of exercise training on the male reproductive system may be comparable to some degree to that found in women. For example, endurance-trained athletes of both sexes have abnormally low levels of the major sex hormones: testosterone in men, and estrogen in women.

The material is divided into four major sections. The first section deals with the basic endocrinology and physiology of testosterone in the male. The second section deals with physiological and methodological issues surrounding the interpretation of research on hormones. The third section covers the changes in testosterone in response to exercise training and acute or prolonged exercise bouts. Finally, in the fourth section the physiological impact of the changes observed in testosterone levels associated with endurance training are discussed.

Basic Endocrinology and Physiology

Testosterone is a steroid hormone. Other steroids in the body include cholesterol, bile acids, vitamin D, and hormones of the adrenal glands and ovary. The majority of circulating testosterone in men comes from production in the interstitial cells of Leydig at the testicles. The adrenal gland also produces small amounts. Regulation of testicular production occurs via a negative feedback loop system involving the anterior pituitary, hypothalamus, and testicles; referred to as the hypothalamic-pituitary-testicular axis. Periodically the hypothalamus releases pulses of gonadotrophin-releasing hormone (GnRH) into the hypophyseal circulation, which supplies the hypothalamus and anterior pituitary. The GnRH stimulates the anterior pituitary to produce and release luteinizing hormone (LH) and follicle-stimulating hormone (FSH).

The pulsatile release of GnRH results in LH and FSH also being released into the systemic circulation in a similar pulsatile manner. For normal, healthy males approximately 2 to 4 LH and FSH pulses are observed over a 6- to 8-hour period, however the amplitudes of the LH pulses are much greater than those observed for FSH. At the testicles, LH and FSH interact with their primary target tissue receptors (LH, Leydig cells; FSH, Sertoli cells) located on the respective cell membranes. Once a hormone-receptor complex is formed, there is an adenyl cyclase-mediated increase of cyclic AMP, which produces a phosphorylation of intracellular proteins by activation of a protein kinase mechanism. In the Leydig cells this protein kinase activation leads to a mobilization of steroid precursors, in particular the activation of pregnenolone synthesis from cholesterol. Pregnenolone serves as the parent compound from which testosterone is derived.

Several other hormones participate in these regulatory events. One worth noting is the anterior pituitary hormone prolactin, which in low concentrations acts as a potentiator of LH at the Leydig cells. Synthesized testosterone diffuses from the Leydig cells into the testicular vascular system and/or into adjacent testicle compartments containing the Sertoli cells. In the Sertoli cells, testosterone plays an essential role in the facilitation of the spermatogenesis process. (The FSH receptor-hormone formation at the Sertoli cell results in the initiation of the spermatogenesis process.)

The pulsatile release of LH results in some fluctuations of testosterone levels in the circulation and additionally there are circadian cycles in which large nocturnal elevations in testosterone can be observed. The majority of the circulating testosterone is transported bound to various carrier proteins (sometimes referred to as binding proteins). The principal carrier protein is sex steroid-binding globulin (SSBG), however other plasma proteins can also bind and carry testosterone to a lesser degree (e.g., albumin, cortisol-binding globulin).

The remaining non-bound circulating testosterone is referred to as free testosterone. This free testosterone is considered the biologically active form of the hormone, as this portion of the hormone can interact at the target tissue receptors. Circulating bound and free testosterone are collectively referred to as total testosterone; sometimes in the literature the term testosterone is used synonymously for total testosterone. Table 1 presents a short summary of the common abbreviations used in this area of endocrinology.

Table 1
Common abbreviations used in reproductive endocrinology as associated with exercise studies and used within this text.

Abbreviation	*Full Name*	*Gland/Tissue of Origin*
T	Testosterone	Testes
LH	Luteinizing hormone	Pituitary
FSH	Follicle stimulating hormone	Pituitary
GnRH	Gonadotrophin-releasing hormone	Hypothalamus
C	Cortisol	Adrenal cortex
SSBG (or SHBG)	Sex steroid-binding globulin (sex hormone-binding globulin)	Liver

Metabolic roles of testosterone

Testosterone has several physiological roles within the male. These roles can be divided into two major categories: androgenic effects, related to reproductive function and the development of a male's secondary sex characteristics, and anabolic effects, pertaining more generally to stimulation of tissue growth.

Androgenic effects: A major reproductive role of testosterone involves the development of the sperm cell. At the Sertoli cells of the testicles, testosterone induces a nuclear activation process which stimulates and catalyses the maturation and development of sperm during the process of spermatogenesis. Maintenance of testosterone levels within the Sertoli cells is essential for the development of adequate numbers of mature, viable sperm that are necessary for a male to be fertile. Testosterone also assists in the development and functioning of the male accessory sex glands (prostate, seminal vesicles, and epididymides), which aid in the sperm development and function, as well as in the act of copulation. Also attributed to the influence of testosterone are the secondary sex characteristics of males, such as the typical deeper male voice, increased levels of body hair, penile growth, sex drive (libido), and more aggressive behavior patterns.

Testosterone also helps red-blood cell development and can produce increased sodium reabsorption in the kidneys. Animal based research has also suggested testosterone plays a role in the increase of tissue glycogen synthesis and storage.

Effectors of testosterone levels

The level of testosterone in the circulation is a function of the amount of hormone entering (testicular production and secretion) and the amount leaving (metabolic clearance) the blood pool. The rates for these processes are affected by any changes in the physiological state that alter metabolic turnover of the hormone.

Production and secretion: Testicular testosterone production in the normal, average male is approximately 7 mg per day. This rate is affected by circulating production stimulators (LH), testicle LH receptor numbers, and synthesis substrate availability.

LH and testosterone levels are directly related. However, it is believed that only a small percentage of the total testicular LH receptors need to be occupied to achieve maximum stimulation of the Leydig cells. Reductions in the numbers of testicular LH receptors can result in reduced levels of testosterone production even in the presence of elevated LH. Receptor numbers can be reduced by certain pathological conditions (e.g. hypergonadotrophic hypogonadism) or a down-receptor phenomena" related state. Persistent elevations in circulating LH can produce a down-regulation of receptor numbers and thereby reduce testicular sensitivity to further changes in blood LH levels.

The conditions of hyperprolactinaemic and hypercortisolemic can also produce lowered testosterone levels. The exact mechanism for this lower testosterone effect is uncertain, but may be due to interference with Leydig cell receptors and/or direct inhibition of the steroidogenic synthesis pathway. Finally, any reduction in availability of steroid hormone precursors (cholesterol, and pregnenolone) can produce a lower rate of testosterone synthesis. Secretion is affected mainly by testicular blood flow through the testicular area, since testosterone is lipid soluble and thus freely diffusible. Furthermore, the testicles apparently have little or no storage capacity for testosterone. Testicular blood flow moreover is a function of the levels of vascular vasoconstriction or vasodilatation. Therefore, anything that influences vascular tone can affect the rate of testosterone secretion.

Metabolic clearance: Testosterone is cleared from the blood by uptake in target tissues and by degradation in the liver. The degradation process involves the conversion of testosterone into 17-ketosteroids and glucuronide, which are excreted into the urine. The hepatic removal process is primarily a function of hepatic blood flow. Thus any changes in the hepatic blood flow can result in concomitant changes in the removal rate of testosterone. Moreover, a small portion of the testosterone is removed from the circulation by select body tissues and then converted to estradiols. It is also important to realize changes observed in blood levels of testosterone may not necessarily reflect alterations in production, secretion, or metabolic clearance rates. A prime example, relative to exercise studies, involves the effect of shifts in plasma. Owing to the binding of testosterone to carrier proteins, increases or decreases in plasma volume lead to a dilution or concentration that is not indicative of changes in the normal hormonal turnover rate. Whether these changes in concentration have a physiological impact is a point of debate.

Methodological Concerns

When discussing factors affecting blood levels of testosterone, consideration must be given to non-physiological factors that could be sources of variation between studies. Examples include blood sampling method, diurnal variations in hormone concentrations, hormone detection methodology, and research protocol. The timing and method of blood sampling are considerations that must be carefully addressed when comparing or evaluating testosterone results of different studies.

The pulsatile release of LH produces fluctuations in the circulating levels of testosterone. Furthermore, as noted earlier there is a daily circadian pattern in blood testosterone levels. A single blood sample will therefore provide an imprecise estimate of the average hormonal level. Use of multiple or serial blood sampling will provide a more accurate assessment. Ideally, the use of a serial method of blood sampling would be preferred and considered more informative of the true status of circulating testosterone. The hormonal biochemical assay methodology must also be considered a source of variability in results. Currently, radioimmunoassays (RIA) are the most common means of assessing testosterone concentrations in blood samples. Since the development of the technique, over 30 years ago, tremendous refinements in procedural and technical aspects have occurred and are still constantly happening. Hence, comparison of hormonal values between studies becomes complicated if a number of years separates the experiments. A comparison problem may also develop if the RIA for the hormone is via a commercial kit versus a laboratory developed technique. In such comparisons, absolute numbers are difficult to contrast directly to one another and the reader must look at relative changes for the most part.

The RIA technique is a relatively easy bioassay to use, as well as inexpensive, and has a high degree of reliability, but there is a limitation: the results represent the immunological activity of the hormone and not necessarily the biological activity. The biological activity depends not only on hormonal levels but also on receptor availability and sensitivity within the individual subject. Finally, examination of the research protocols of studies that compare the hormonal status of exercising and non-exercising subjects reveals several problems. For example, to examine the effects of endurance training most studies have compared aerobically trained men with untrained sedentary-control men, in a retrospective fashion.

The problem with this approach is the trained men have subjected themselves to the rigors of the training program, typically for years and the investigator is observing the end result. Because of the wide variations in response to training, as well as variations in the exact type of training, considerable divergence can be observed in the testosterone responses of these subjects. Another problem develops from the large discrepancy in what individual authors define as exercise training and exercise-trained states. For example, some researchers may consider an individual as chronically trained if they have performed regular exercise for one year, while other research may indicate that a five-year period is necessary. Additionally, one of the principal assumptions made within these retrospective studies is that the observed effects on testosterone levels are the results of the exercise training performed by the subject. Obviously, this assumption is not valid unless such things as psychological stresses, sleep loss, diet, weight loss, and hereditary factors, all of which affect testosterone level, are controlled.

Exercise and Testosterone

The results of the retrospective comparative studies examining isolated, single blood samples suggest lower testosterone levels in chronically endurance-trained males. The subjects in these studies have typically been distance runners who had been involved with the physical training aspects of their sport for 1 to 15 years. In these studies, testosterone levels of the endurance-trained men were found to be 60-85% of the levels of matched, untrained men. Prospective studies have also been conducted in which blood samples have been collected over days or weeks while exposing subjects to endurance training regimens. Findings thus far have been inconsistent, as some reports reveal significant reductions in resting testosterone following 1 to 6 months of intensive training, while others found no significant resting testosterone changes after 2 to 3 months of training. Differences in the initial training status of the subjects or the training administered may explain these discrepancies.

Endurance-trained males with lower testosterone also display other reproductive hormonal abnormalities. The most frequently reported changes involve decreased resting levels of prolactin and more importantly, no significant elevations in resting LH, even though there is decreased testosterone. These findings of altered prolactin and LH levels at rest in endurance trained men with low testosterone have been labeled by some researchers as a dysfunction of the hypothalamic-pituitary-testicular (HPT) regulatory axis. These findings with prolactin and LH have been reported in retrospective and prospective studies. Several investigators have also conducted retrospective investigations where resting blood samples were collected every 20 or 30 min for 4- to 8-hour periods from chronically endurance-trained men and untrained controls. Results are similar to those of the isolated-sampling studies: resting testosterone concentration of the trained subjects were typically 70-80% of those found in the controls. As with isolated blood sampling studies, resting LH levels have not been significantly elevated. Again, these findings have been cited as a dysfunction in the HPT axis. These studies have been performed mainly with endurance runners, but it is likely that the effects apply to endurance athletes generally. Mechanisms of HPT Axis Dysfunction. Several studies have attempted to elucidate the mechanism of the proposed HPT axis dysfunction found in endurance-trained men. These studies have focused on examining whether the dysfunction is central (hypothalamic or pituitary) or peripheral (testicular).

Centrally, the research work has focused upon alterations in LH release and/or prolactin release. Alterations in LH and prolactin release have been an area of extensive research relative to the study of exercising women who develop reproductive dysfunction. An exaggerated prolactin release to an exogenous stimulus of drugs or synthetic hormones has been found in endurance-trained males with low testosterone. Conversely, an attenuated release of LH due to doses of GnRH has been detected in endurance-trained males. Prolactin presents an interesting paradox in reproductive physiological function. Small amounts of prolactin seem necessary to work synergistically at the testicle with LH, while excessive levels disrupt both central and peripheral aspects of the HPT axis.

Several investigators have found this altered prolactin and LH release. Interestingly, although overall LH response is decreased, results are contradictory as to whether LH pulsatile characteristics (i.e., pulse frequency and amplitude) are affected by endurance training.

Peripherally, alterations in the sensitivity of the testes to LH changes has been the key research focus. Evaluations of testicular sensitivity to an exogenous stimulus have shown trained and untrained males to have comparable responses. Thus, these overall findings would suggest the development of a central problem in the HPT axis; however, data in this area are limited and not yet definitive. An acute exercise bout could induce transient increases in circulating prolactin and cortisol, which could account for the observed changes in testosterone.

The likelihood, however, of either of these transient states being a causative factor is doubtful. These are relatively small, temporary changes in prolactin and cortisol levels in response to exercise. Generally, the lowered testosterone associated with increased prolactin or cortisol is due to chronic supra-physiological elevations of these hormones that usually result from pathological states such as pituitary or adrenal tumors.

Changes in response to exercise

It is generally accepted that short-term maximal exercise results in an elevation of circulation testosterone levels. It is still an issue of some debate whether this effect is due simply to hemoconcentration effects, reduced metabolic clearance and/or possibly a hormone-mediated increase in testicular production. Surprisingly few studies have performed direct comparisons of exercise testosterone responses between endurance-trained (with low testosterone levels) and untrained control men. There appear to be no major differences in response between the two types of subject, but this area is in need of further investigation. Typically testosterone responses to submaximal exercise are somewhat variable and seem dependent on the duration and intensity of exercise. A progressive increase in testosterone occurs during moderate exercise lasting 45 to 90 minutes, but 90 minutes of submaximal exercise has also been reported to produce no change or slight decreases in testosterone concentration. Exercise of a moderate to hard intensity performed until exhaustion or of more than 2 hours duration results in lowered testosterone concentrations. These changes in testosterone during submaximal exercise may be due to the interaction of several factors. Initially with submaximal exercise, hemoconcentration may produce elevations in testosterone levels. However, as the exercise continues there are reductions in testicular production and secretion.

These production/secretion reductions appear to be principally the effects of declining testicular blood flow. Concurrently with the reduced testicle blood flow, hepatic blood flow may also be compromised, resulting in a declining hepatic clearance, which may further elevate testosterone levels. This latter change may be offset by an increased uptake by skeletal muscle as exercise duration continues, resulting in gradual reduction in testosterone levels. The acute effects of maximal and submaximal exercise on testosterone levels last a relatively short period of time (~1 to 48 hours). Again, few studies seem to have compared submaximal exercise testosterone responses between endurance-trained (with low testosterone levels) and untrained control men. There is no evidence to suggest extensive response differences between the two types of subjects.

Physiological impact of lower testosterone

Currently, there is little evidence to suggest that the development of low resting testosterone levels in men doing endurance training has any major detrimental effect on the testosterone-dependent physiological processes of the body. There is the potential for disruption in any of the processes influenced by testosterone, and obviously reproductive capacity is of key concern. Few studies have systematically studied this issue and currently only a few reports of decreased spermatogenesis or oligospermatic conditions existing in endurance trained males have been published.

Additionally, some investigators have reported endurance trained men may have a lowered sex drive; but a direct cause-and-effect linkage between a lower sex drive and testosterone did not exist in these data. There are also apparently no significant detrimental effects of lower testosterone on the other anabolic-androgenic effects of testosterone (protein synthesis and muscle mass development). However, this area has not been examined thoroughly by the exercise science community. An additional area in need of research concerns bone demineralization and low testosterone. Clinically, there is strong evidence indicating hypogonadal and hypo-testosteronemic men have severe mineral loss from their bones. There are no conclusive findings of mineral content change in endurance trained men with low testosterone, but several compelling case studies have been reported in the literature.

On the other hand, there could be beneficial physiologic adaptations from the lowered testosterone. Some researchers indicate that lowering testosterone may have cardiovascular protective effects and decrease the risk of coronary heart disease. A recent study out of Germany has provided strong evidence supporting this claim. This research has demonstrated that chemically induced reductions in endogenous testosterone level results in significant increases in high-density lipoprotein in men. Whether the lowering of testosterone in men performing endurance training will produce the same effect remains to be determined.

Endurance exercise training would seem to have significant effects upon the major male reproductive hormone, testosterone. A growing body of evidence suggests at rest testosterone is lowered in the endurance-trained male. The mechanism of this lowering is currently unclear, but may be related to dysfunction within the HPT regulatory axis brought about by months or years of endurance training. Currently, the time course of the changes in the reproductive endocrine system are unresolved. There are only limited findings to indicate that endurance training disrupts testosterone-dependent anabolic or androgenic processes in the male. The alterations in testosterone levels brought by endurance exercise training could even have cardiovascular protective effects.

Jet-Lag Symptoms and Treatment

The feelings of disorientation encountered as a result of crossing time zones are known as jet lag. Symptoms include fatigue and general tiredness, inability to sleep at night, loss of concentration, loss of drive, headaches and general malaise. Jet-lag occurs when biological rhythms are disrupted as a result of rapid transitions across multiple time-zones. Such desynchronization of rhythms also occurs in nocturnal shift work employees who transfer to night shifts. A classical rhythm is represented by a sine wave, fluctuations occurring cyclically about a mean value rising to a peak and half a cycle later dropping to a trough. Twenty-four hour rhythms are known as circadian (about a day). An example of a biological rhythm is core temperature. We can find the characteristics of rhythms using the mathematical technique of cosinor analysis to determine the mean, the peak, the amplitude, and the time the peak occurs (the acrophase).

Circadian Desynchronization

Following a journey across multiple time zones the body's rhythms at first retain the characteristics of their point of departure. However, the new environment forces new influences on these cycles, the main factors being the time of sunrise and onset of darkness. The body attempts to adjust to this new context but core temperature is relatively sluggish in doing so. As a rough guide it takes about one day for each time zone crossed for body temperature to adapt completely.

The individual may have difficulty in sleeping for a few days, but activity and social contact during the day help in accelerating the adaptations of the arousal rhythm. Thus arousal adjusts more quickly than does body temperature to the new time zone. Until the whole spectrum of biological rhythms adjusts to the new local time, the performance of exercise may be below par. Allowing for individual differences, the severity of jet lag is affected by a variety of factors. In general, the greater the number of time zones crossed, the more difficult it is to cope.

A 2-hour phase shift may have marginal significance but a 3-hour shift (e.g. British or Irish teams traveling to play European football matches in Russia or Turkey or a Californian sports team traveling to play on the east coast of the US) will entail desynchronization to a substantial degree. In such cases the flight times time of departure and time of arrival - may determine the severity of symptoms. The severity of symptoms may be worse 2-3 days after arrival than on the day immediately following disembarkation.

Symptoms then gradually abate, but can still be acute at particular times of day. There will be a window of time during the day when the period of high arousal associated with the time zone just left overlaps with the arousal high point at the new local time. This window may be predicted in advance and should be utilized for timing of training practices in the first few days at destination. Our observations on footballers traveling from Britain to the South Pacific indicate that morning training sessions suit players best over the first few days. Such a practice has also proved successful for cross-country runners. The direction of travel affects the severity of jet lag. It is easier to cope with flying in a westward direction compared to flying eastward. In flying westward the normal cycle is temporarily lengthened and body rhythms can extend in line with their natural freewheeling period of about 27 hours and thus catch up. Observations on traveling to Korea (9 hours in advance of British Summer time) and Malaysia (7 hours in advance of British Summer time) are that periods of 9 and 6 days respectively may be inadequate for jet lag symptoms to disappear. In contrast re-adaptation is more rapid on returning to Britain. When time zone shifts approach the maximum 12-hour change, there may be little difference between eastward and westward travel. The direction of travel can be a relevant consideration when going from coast to coast to compete in North America. When going eastward the mean performance is depressed more and the peak performance declines more dramatically than is the case on traveling westward.

The reason for westward travel being easier is because the natural period of circadian rhythms is greater than 24 hours, so each rhythm adapts more quickly when the day is artificially lengthened. Altering training times for a few days prior to travel to take into consideration the time of competition in another time zone is known to be beneficial. Young individuals have a better tolerance to desynchronization of rhythms, owing to a better regulation of biological clocks.

Physical fitness also seems to play a role: active subjects demonstrate higher amplitudes in existing rhythms than age-matched controls, a difference indicative of superior regulation. But other than these factors, there has been little success in attempting to predict good and poor adapters to long haul flights. Furthermore, the fact that an individual escapes lightly from symptoms on one occasion is no guarantee that he or she will do so again on the next visit.

Reducing Jet Lag

If it is possible to do so, flights should be scheduled so that athletes arrive well in advance of competition. One day for each time zone crossed does leave a cushion of safety, even traveling eastward. The time for adaptation may be shortened by exploiting the external factors that reset biological clocks: rest/exercise, darkness/ light, meals and social influences. The key is to tune in straight away to the external influences of the new environment. It may be beneficial to shop around to find the most convenient travel schedules. Consider departure from regional airports if appropriate and also alternative carriers. The routines prior to departure, on the plane, and after arrival, can be planned once the itinerary is established. In consequence coping with jet lag will not be the hit or miss affair it might otherwise be.

On lengthy journeys it is unlikely that any maneuvers will eliminate jet lag, but with careful planning the symptoms can be attenuated. In the week prior to departure it may be possible to adjust the time of arising and going to bed, the adjustment depending on the direction of flight. An alteration of more than two hours is likely to be unproductive, since this would interfere with the pattern of social and domestic engagements during the day. Besides, the major synchronizer of human circadian rhythms--natural daylight--remains unaltered. The evidence from simply altering time of retiring to sleep is that shifting the sleep-wake cycle does alter rhythms in accord with the direction of the shift, but motor performance is compromised during the course of such adaptive changes. Manipulating the sleep-wakefulness rhythm prior to traveling abroad to compete therefore may not be the best strategy. Once flight times are known, a routine on the plane may be planned. In day time flights it will be necessary to stay awake, keep mentally active and perhaps watch the in-flight movie. On long haul flights that entail traveling during the night it will be necessary to get some sleep on the plane.

The timing of this should be decided in advance so that some meals on board can be missed. Transit or transfer episodes en route should be taken into consideration. It is a good strategy to set one's watch to local time at the next point of landing, once on board the plane: in a single haul flight this would be the local time of the country of destination. The important thing is that the traveler mentally tunes in to the new local time straight away and adjusts behavior accordingly. To compensate for the dry air on board flight, copious rehydration is advised. Fruit juices are best, fizzy drinks should be avoided. Alcohol should not be taken, since it acts as a diuretic (increases urine production) and also affects the normal circadian rhythm in renal function.

Caffeine in coffee also stimulates water loss, and its arousal effect on the central nervous system means it should not be taken if sleep is desired. One suggestion is that the last meal prior to the time allotted for sleep should be high in carbohydrates and low in protein in order to induce drowsiness. Carbohydrates provide the substrate for serotonin, a neurotransmitter that regulates sleep. Caffeine and a low-carbohydrate high-protein breakfast would help raise the level of arousal and prevent a relapse into sleep.Athletes may feel stiff or cramped because of their restrained posture on board flight. They can perform isometric exercises for arms, trunk or legs while in their seats. It is even better to walk down the aisle of the plane and occasionally do flexibility or stretching exercises at the back of the plane. British sports teams traveling to Australia have used sleeping pills to induce sleep while on board. Although such drugs as benzodiazepines are effective in getting people to sleep, they do not guarantee a prolonged period asleep. Besides, they have not been satisfactorily tested for subsequent residual effects on motor performances such as sports skills. They may also be counter-productive if administered at the incorrect time. A prolonged nap at the time the individual feels drowsy (presumably at the time that he or she would have been asleep in the time zone departed from) simply anchors the rhythms at their former phases and so resists the adaptations to the new time zone.

On reaching the country of destination a key factor is to fit in immediately with the phase characteristics of the new environment. Athletes should already have worked out the local time for their disembarkation. There may be other environmental factors to consider such as heat, humidity or even altitude. Having traveled westward, players may be allowed to retire to bed early. Early onset of sleep will be less likely after an eastward flight. In this case a light training session on that evening would be helpful in instilling local cues into the rhythms. Besides, there is some evidence that exercise does speed up the adaptation to a new time zone. For the first few days in the new time zone, training sessions should not be all-out efforts. Skills requiring fine co-ordination are likely to be impaired and this might lead to accidents or injuries if, for example, games players conducted sessions with the ball too strenuously. Where a series of tournament engagements is scheduled, it is useful to have at least one friendly match during the initial period in the overseas country.

In this period of adaptation a few caveats are noted. Alcohol taken late in the evening is likely to disrupt sleep and so is not advised. The alternation of feasting and fasting recommended for commercial travelers in the USA is unlikely to gain acceptance among footballers. Nevertheless they could benefit from biasing the macronutrients in their evening meal largely towards carbohydrates. These would include vegetables with a choice of chipped, roast or baked potatoes, pasta dishes, rice and bread. These should include sufficient fiber to safeguard against constipation. In the early days in the new country athletes should be discouraged from taking prolonged naps.

A nap at the time they would have been asleep had they stayed at home would make subsequent sleep more difficult and retard the adjustment of the major biological clocks to the new regimens. Exposure to bright light, preferably natural daylight, is a useful antidote to drowsiness in such circumstances. Taking drugs can alter biological clocks, depending on the time they are taken. Caffeine (in coffee) and theophylline (in tea) are stimulantsm of the central nervous system. Taken in the evening they would help in recovery after flying eastward and in the afternoon after flying westward. The minor tranquilizers, benzodiaepines, affect neurotransmitters that have a role in arousal. These include serotonin, noradrenaline, acetylcholine and gamma-aminobutyric acid (GABA). As already indicated, they are effective in inducing sleep but not necessarily good in ensuring the state of sleep. Also hangover effects cannot be excluded, even in some so-called short-acting hypnotics.

Administration of melatonin, which is a pineal gland hormone, has shown good results in treating Scandinavian patients suffering depression in the winter. This clinical condition is known as seasonal affective disorder. The lack of stimulus from natural light for the pineal gland to secrete melatonin is a recognized cause of this entity. Prolonged exposure to bright artificial light has also proved effective in those patients. Subjects who took melatonin tablets on a trip from Britain to Australia experienced a reduction in jet-lag symptoms, improvements in sleep quality, and a faster readjustment of cortisol and melatonin rhythms. These findings received further support from results of a simulated eastward flight across nine time zones. It seems that administration of melatonin in the afternoon or evening causes phase advances of circadian rhythms whereas a phase delay (required after a westward flight) results from administration at night or early morning. However, toxic side-effects of this substance cannot be discounted and besides, it is not yet readily available in tablet form. There is also a suggestion that the amino acid tryptophan is helpful in coping with jet-lag. It is a precursor of the sleep hormones, but there is no evidence that it improves the quality of sleep. Besides, it has achieved bad publicity in the early 1990s due to impurities being found in commercially available products and its use is no longer recommended.

It is more effective to use light or behavioral measures to resynchronize circadian rhythms. Natural daylight and bright artificial light help to increase or maintain arousal as well as contribute to returning endogenous rhythms. For athletes exercise is a powerful resynchronizor. It stimulates catecholamines and alertness. It is recommended, even on the day of arrival, except late in the evening local time. Exercise at a light intensity is adequate for stimulating resynchronization of rhythmic characteristics as exercise that is too strenuous may disrupt rather than promote sleep.

Bibliography

Andreasen J.O, and F.M. Andreasen, *Essentials of Traumatic Injuries to the Teeth*, Munksgaard Publishing, 1991, pp11-12.

American Dental Association, *Council on Dental Materials*, Mouth Protectors and Sports Team Dentists. JADA 1984;109:84- 87.

Bailey D, "Physical Activity and the Attainment of Peak Bone Mass in Children", *The Australian Journal of Science and Medicine in Sport*, 26 March/June 94 (1/2) : 3 - 5

Duda M., *Which Athletes Should Wear Mouthguards? The Physician and Sports Medicines*, Vol 15, No 9, September 87.

Handler, SD, "Diagnosis and Management of Maxillofacial Injuries", *Chapter 40; Torg J.S., Athletic Injuries to the Head, Neck, and Face; Mosby Year Book*, 1991, pp611-613.

Hardcourt, J.K., Aust. *Dent Journal*, 1989:34:5 pp485.

Hickey, Judson C, Morris, Alvin L, Carlson, Loren D., Seward, Thomas E., "The Relation of Mouth Protectors to Cranial Pressure and Deformation", *JADA*, Vol.74, March 1967.

Padilla R, Dorney B, Balikov S, "Mouthguards-Prevention of Oral Injuries", *Journal California Dental Association*, March 1996, Vol 24, No.3.

Park et al, "Methods of Improved Mouthguards", *First International Symposium on Biomaterials*, Taejon, Korea, August 1993.

Pinkham J R, Kohn D W "Epidemiology and Prediction of Sports Related Traumatic Injuries", *Dental Clinics of America*, Vol 35, No 4, October 1991, pp 609-625.

Tavener M, Payne W "The Effects of Participation in a 'Health of Primary Schools Program' on the Physical Fitness of Children" *The Australian Journal of Science and Medicine in Sport*, September 1993 25 (3):84-85.

Torg, J.S., *Athletic Injuries to the Head, Neck, and Face*, 2nd ed., Mosby Year Book, 1991., pg.611-612.

Ranalli, DN, "Prevention of Craniofacial Injuries in Football", *The Dental Clinics of North America*, Sports Dentistry; Vol 35, No.4, Oct.1991, Saunders, pp635.

Stenger J.M., "Mouthguards: Protection Against Shock to Head Neck and Teeth", *JADA* 1964, 69:273-281.

Stenger, John M, "Physiologic Dentistry with Notre Dame Players", *Basal Facts*, Spring, 1977;2(1):8-18

Index